Meditations on Motherhood

J.K. COLLINS

with illustrations by Emilee Hanks

REPUTATION BOOKS

MEDITATIONS ON MOTHERHOOD

Published by Reputation Books, LLC
www.reputationbooksllc.com

Cover and book design: Lisa Abellera
Cover art and illustrations © Emilee Hanks

ISBN 978-1-944387-19-8

First Edition: April 2021

10 9 8 7 6 5 4 3 2 1

Reputation Books

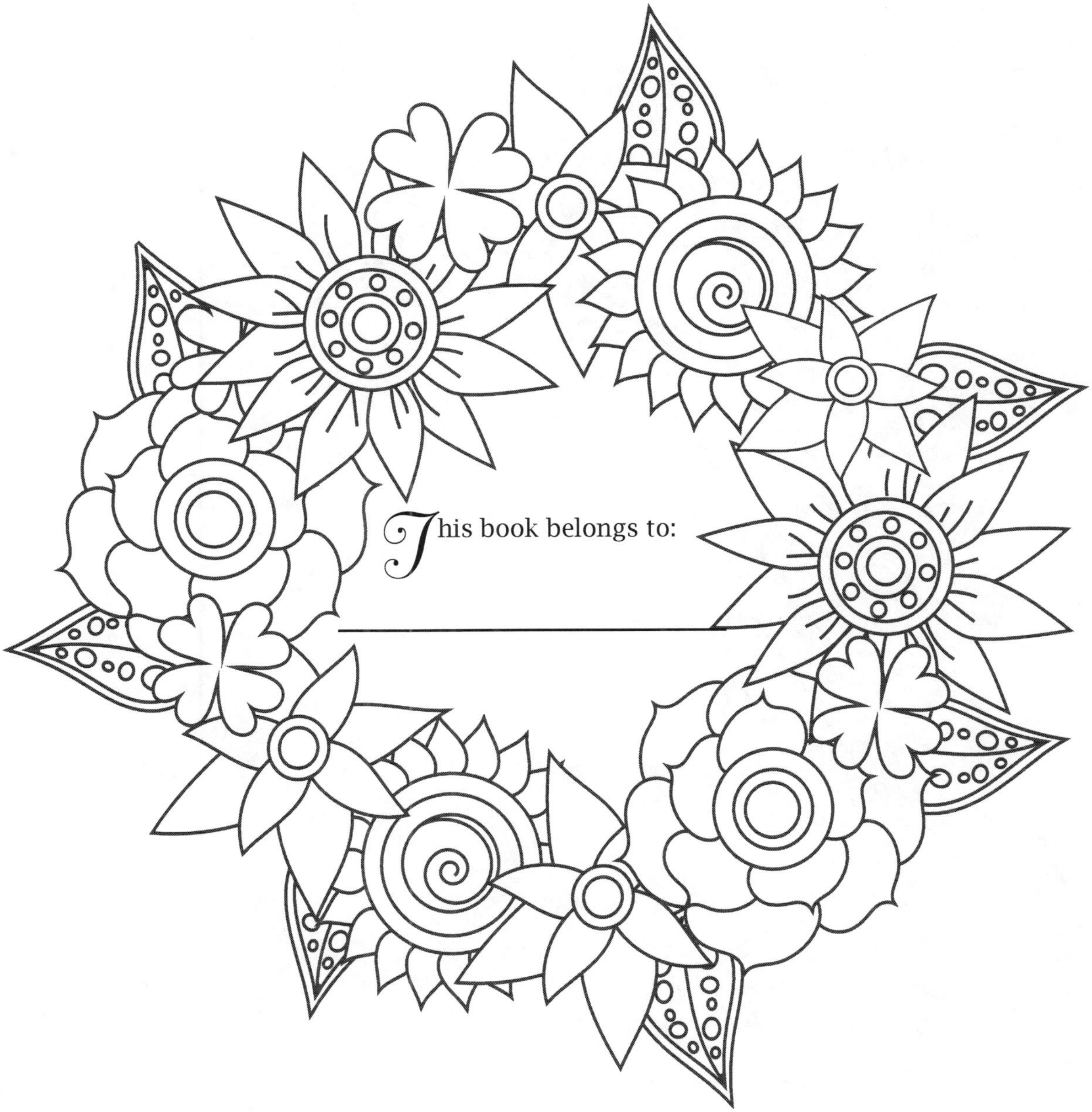

This book belongs to:

____

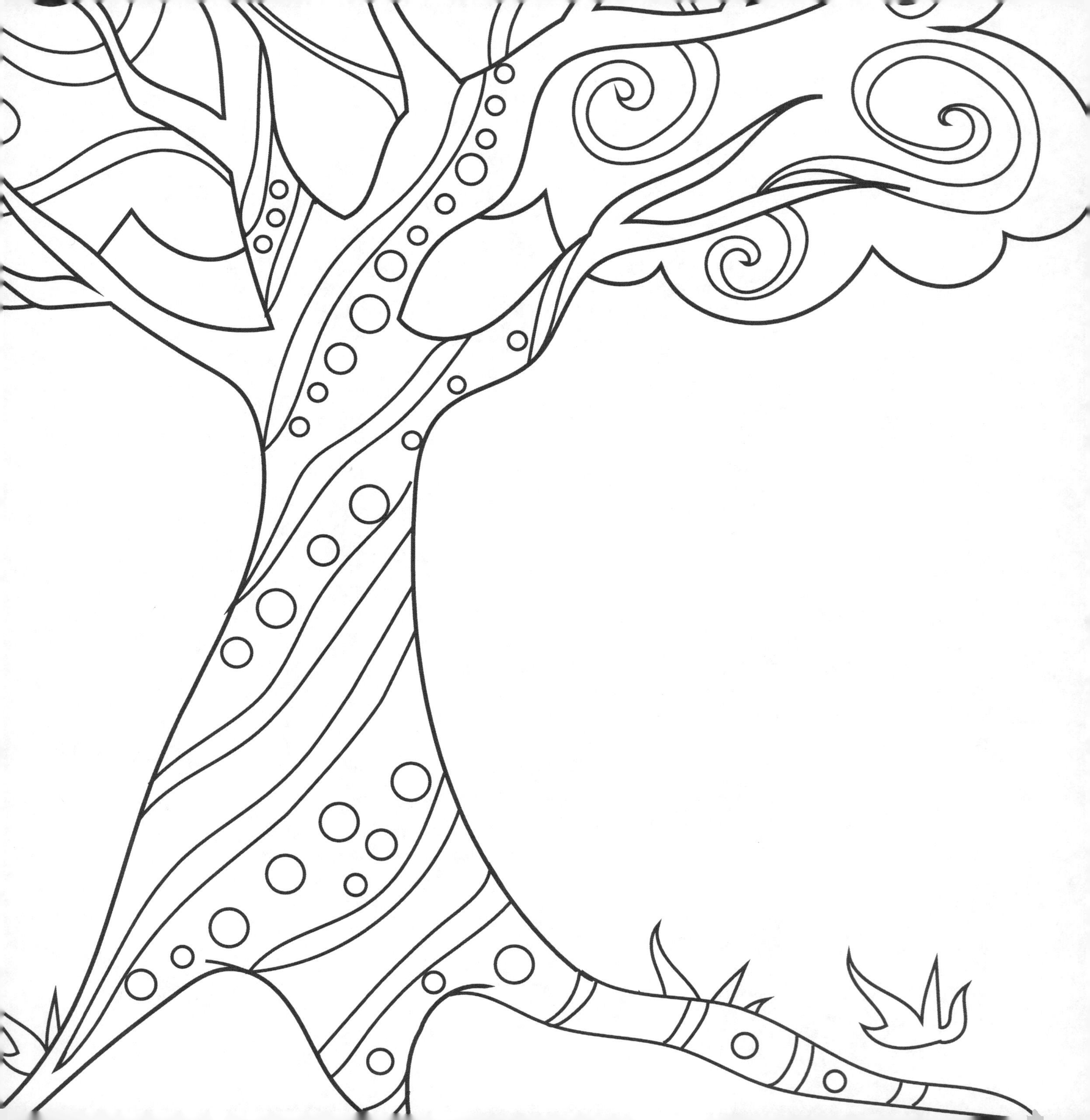

Motherhood is a special privilege that women share, whether it's by giving birth or raising a child in any capacity. Motherhood is based on love, giving unconditionally, and reaping the benefits of smiles, affection, and lasting relationships on this earth.

I write this book of meditations, hopeful that by reflecting on the extraordinary blessings that touch our lives through our children we are able to pause, take a breath, and appreciate the gifts—as well as responsibilities—that accompany Motherhood. May this book inspire and celebrate what you have given of yourself, and help you appreciate the sacred journey that continues throughout your life.

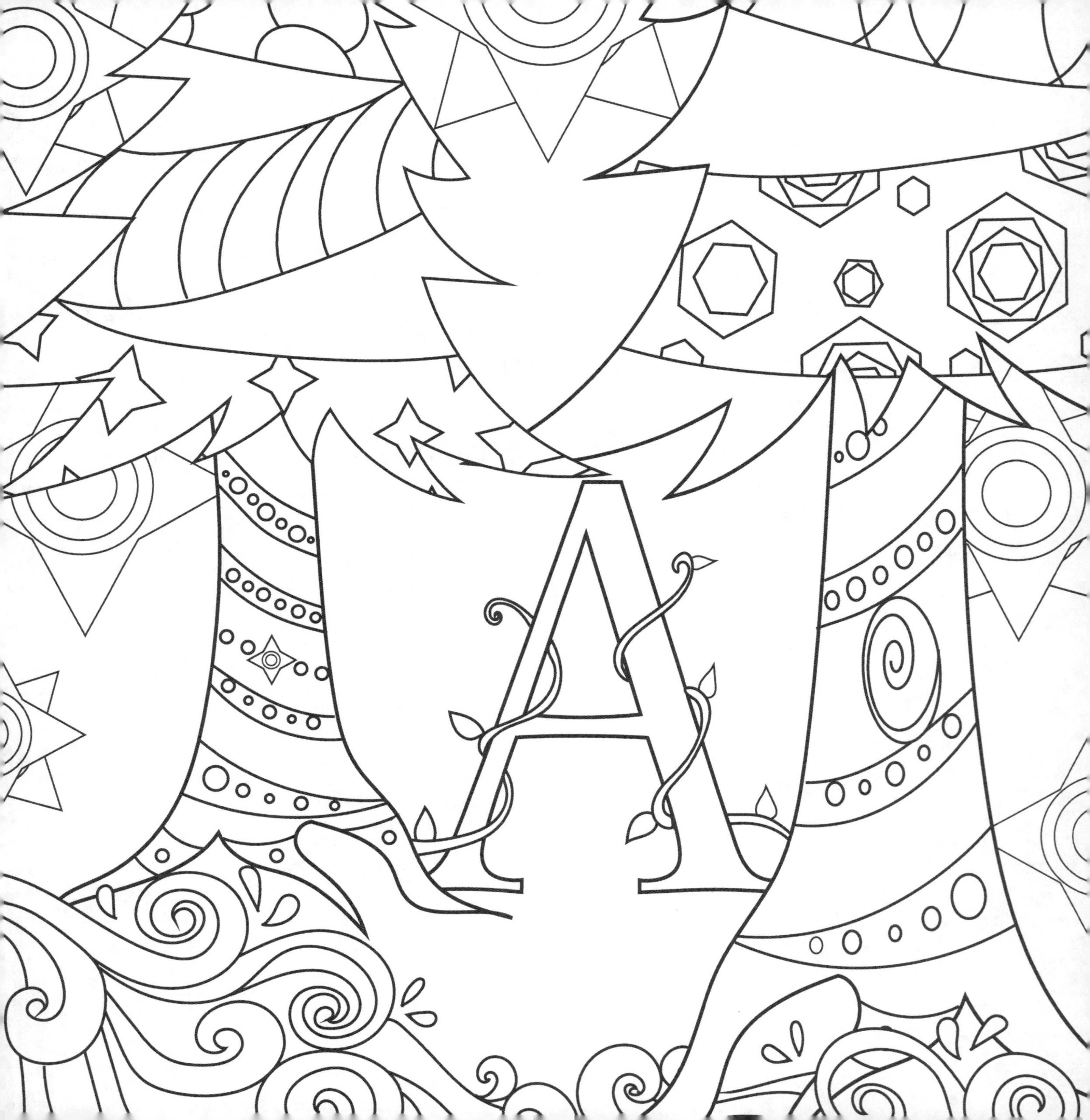
A

A is for ACCOMODATING. . . .

We, as Mothers, learn quickly to be flexible and accommodating to a child's needs. We ADJUST our lives to make sure our children are healthy and happy, as much as possible. ACCOMPANYING our children wherever they go, we give them our time, our love, and our hearts as we nurture and protect them.

ADAPTING ourselves to their needs, we learn that those come first, and ACCLIMATE our lives to provide the ATTENTION, as well as love that they require.

When our children are healthy and happy, we feel ACCOMPLISHED. We are often tested during times of ADOLESCENCE, but learn patience and flexibility.

If we consistently give them the unconditional love they need, their ADMIRATION grows and we earn their love and respect. We ADORE our children, and hope to give them the best years of our lives. We always have AFFECTION

Breathe in ACCEPTANCE. . . . Breathe out ABSOLUTION. . . .

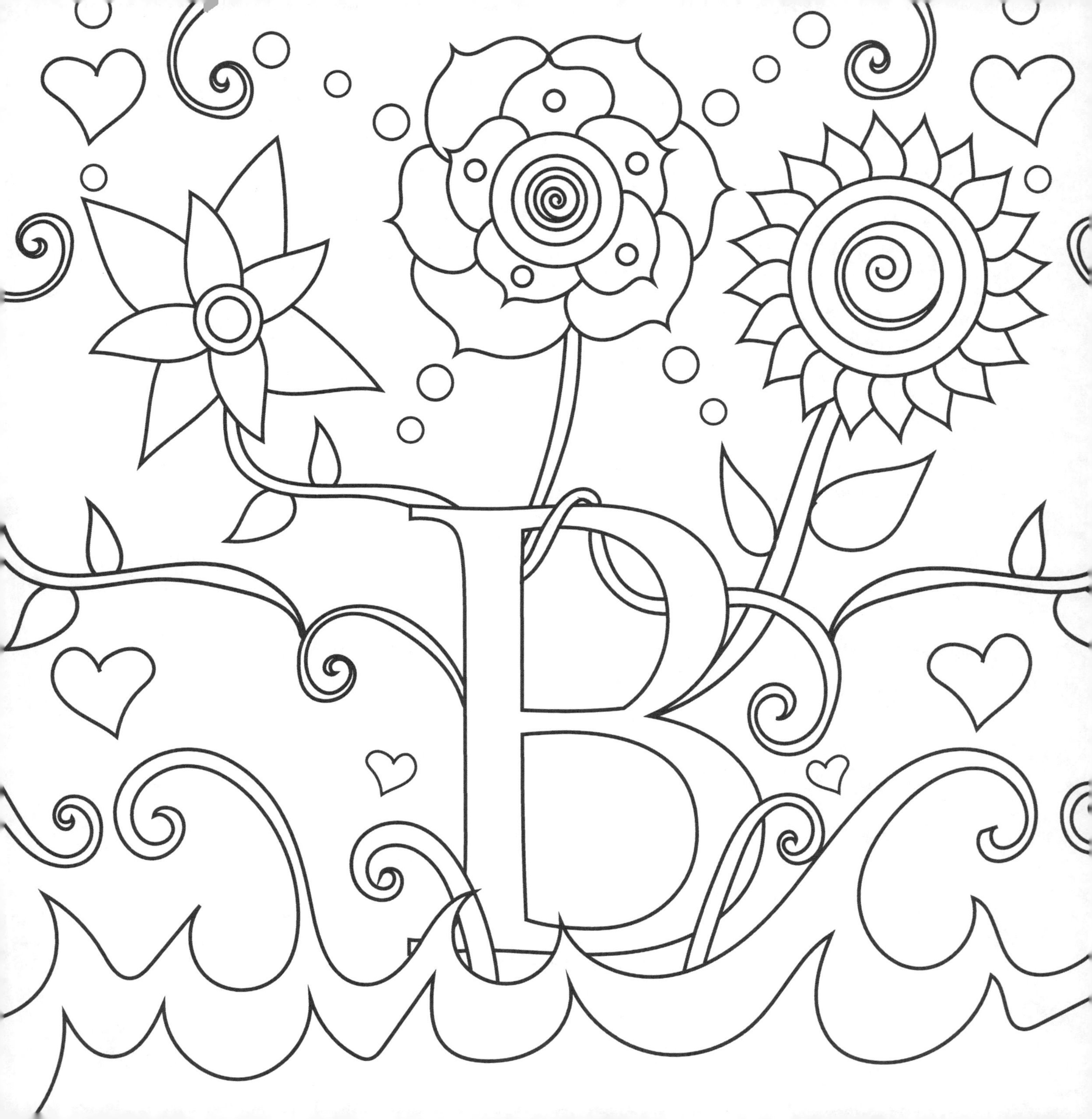
B

B is for BOUNTIFUL. . . .

Our lives become so enriched as we experience the privilege of Motherhood. The joy and laughter of BABIES delights us, and we realize how responsible we must be to take care of them.

We learn to BALANCE our lives and those of our children by making BOUNDARIES. We hope to lessen their BURDENS in life by introducing them to BOOKS.

They forever keep us BUSY, as we BUY the food and clothes that nurture and keep them warm. We are often BAFFLED by their wit and reactions, and we BEAM with love over their achievements.

We hope to teach them not to be BIASED in their opinions and perspectives, and to think for themselves, always. We BEGIN again, to grow in ways that we never thought possible.

Breathe in BEAUTY. . . . Breathe out BLESSINGS. . . .

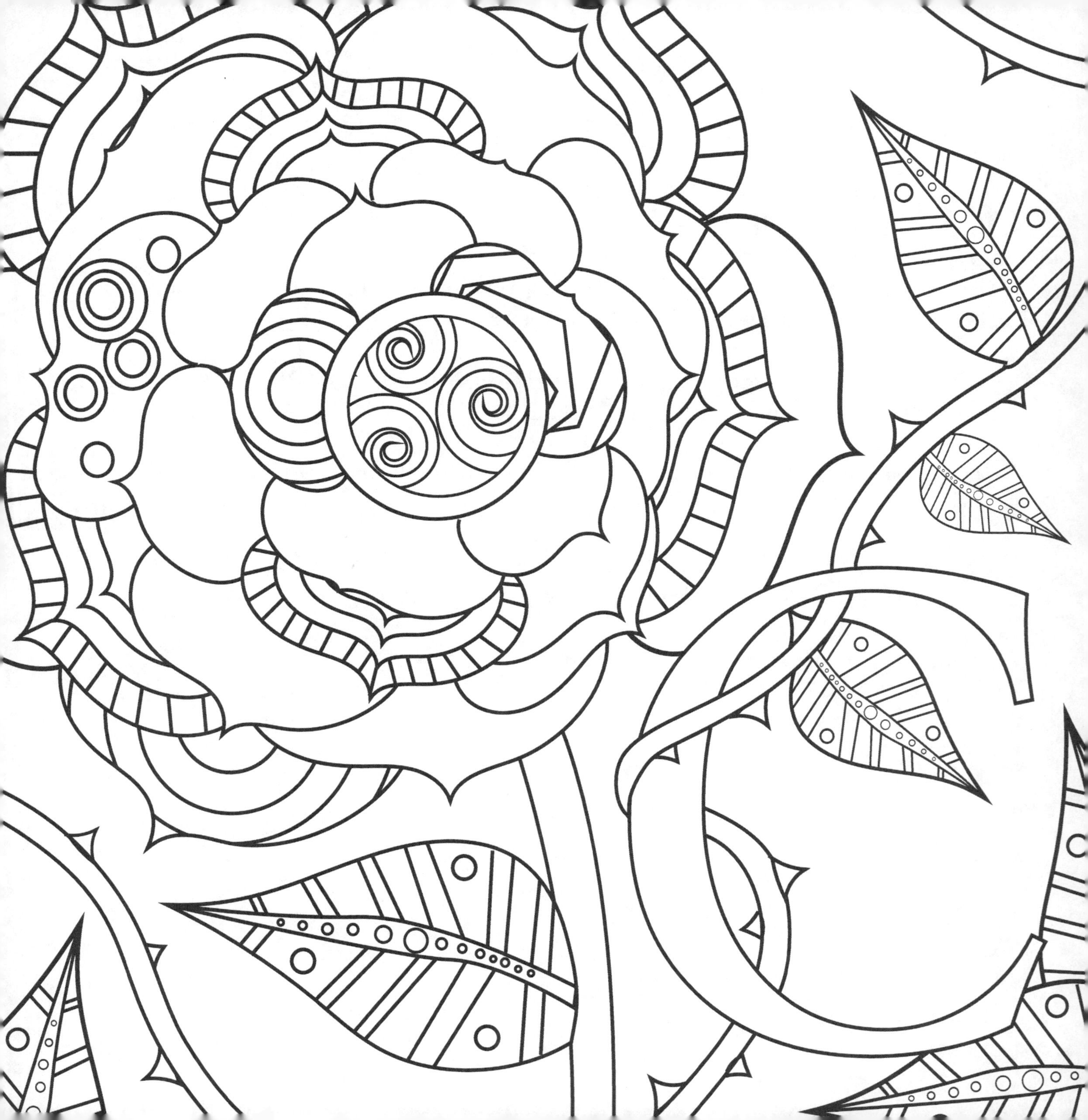

C is for CHILDHOOD. . . . .

We are the CUSTODIANS of CHILDREN'S lives, and nurture them to grow into COMFORTABLE, responsible adults. We CARE for them with CONCERN for their well-being.

We CATER to their needs, and COMMUNICATE our love, as well as our COUNCIL. A Mother COACHES and CALMS her children. We CUDDLE them and CULTIVATE their talents and abilities to be CIVILIZED in their behavior towards others.

We CELEBRATE their happy moments, their birthdays, as well as their CONTRADICTIONS.

We hope to teach them good COMMUNICATION skills so they may truly hear others. Throughout our lives, we are their CHAMPIONS.

Breathe in CHARITY. . . . Breathe out CONFIDENCE. . . .

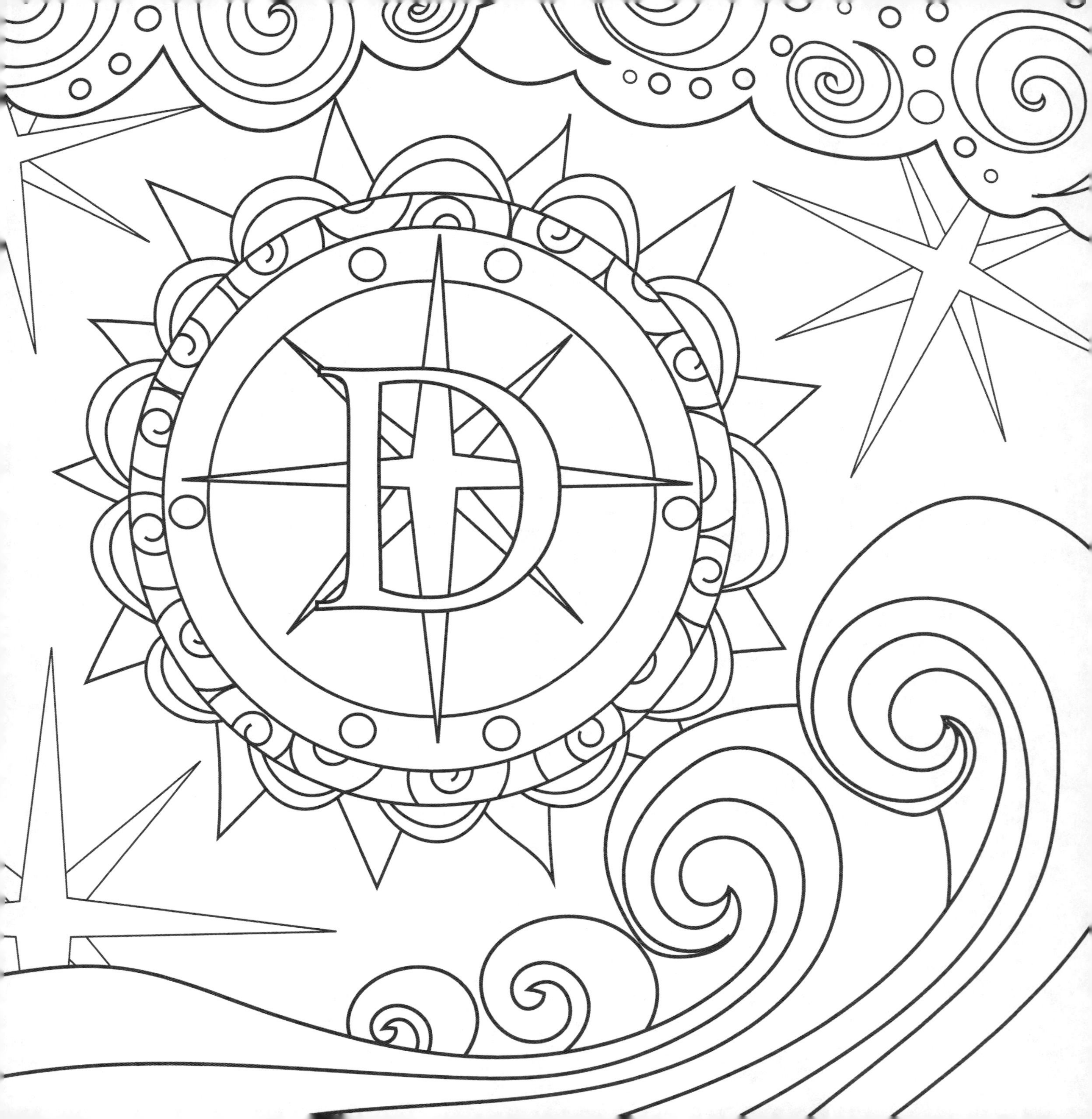
D

D is for DETERMINATION. . . .

Our children are our DIVINE gifts—they offer us DIFFERENT and unique perspectives in seeing the world through their eyes.

They are our DARLINGS. We help them learn to make the right DECISIONS in their lives, and they teach us DILIGENCE.

The DREAMS we have for our children stay with us always, but whatever they choose in life, it is their DESTINATION, not ours that DETERMINES their choices.

We must remember to DWELL in their happiness, whatever choices they make. Our DHARMA is to let go and let them live their own lives, however DIFFICULT it is.

Breathe in DHARMA. . . . Breathe out DIVINITY. . . .

E is for ENERGY. . . .

EVERYDAY, our children bring us joy. During their EARLY years, our job is to make sure they are healthy and happy. We EDUCATE them with the lessons of life.

We watch their EFFORTS, as they struggle to learn to walk, ride bikes, and make relationships. We are EFFUSIVE with our love for them, and listen to them with EMPATHY.

We are miserable when we feel their suffering, and ELATED when they succeed. A Mother must learn to EMBRACE change, as our children grow to live independently of us.

Our children ENLIGHTEN and ENTICE us to ENGAGE with their lives. We ENVELOPE them with our love and wisdom, hoping to EMBELLISH their lives.

We hope to teach them a sense of ELEGANCE.

Breathe in ENLIGHTENMENT. . . . Breathe out EMPATHY. . . .

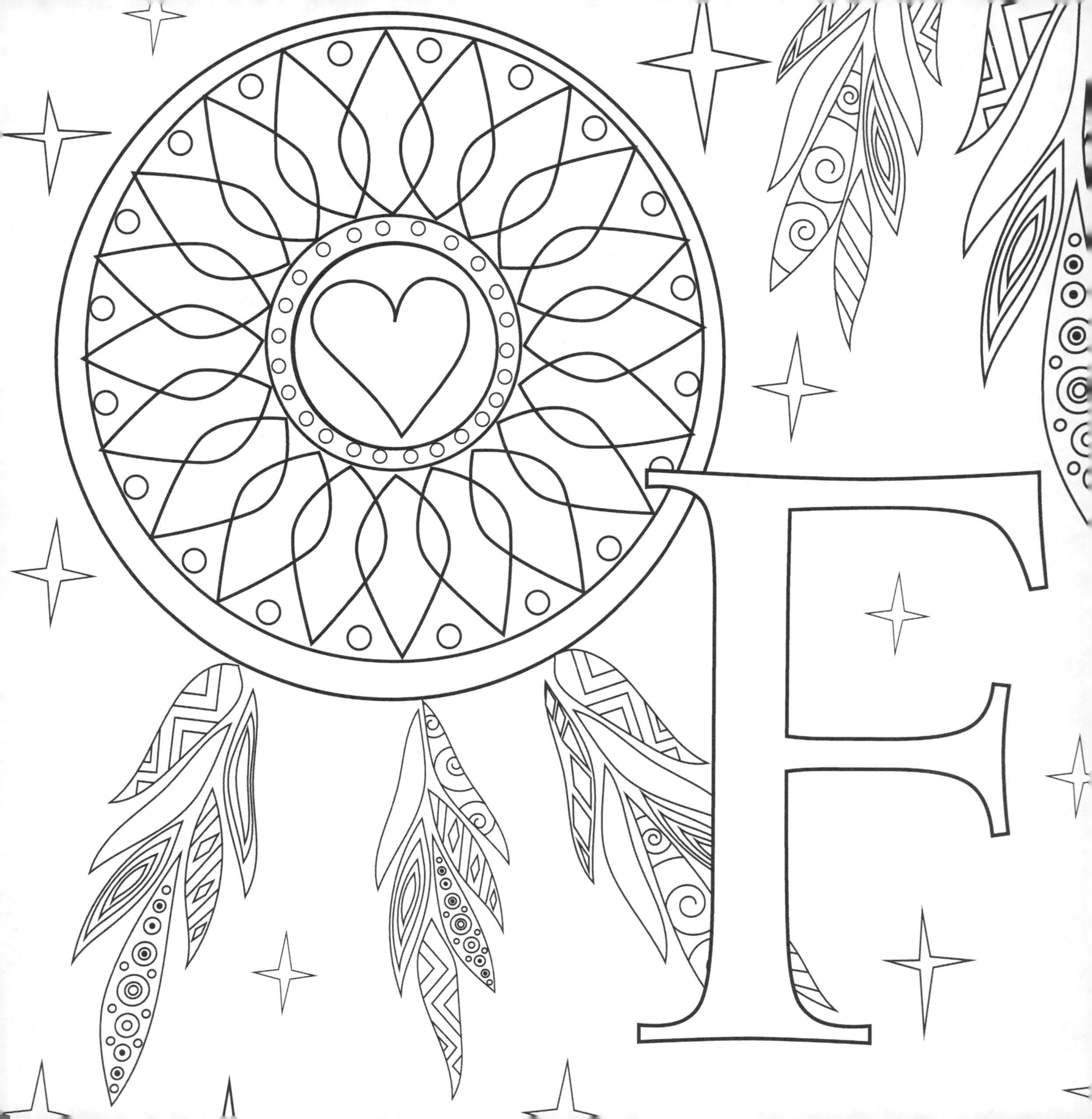
F

F is for FAMILY. . . .

By FORGING our relationships, we FINALLY make a choice as to whom we would like to raise a family with. FOLLOWING our instincts, we make a choice with a partner that we hope is FOREVER. FINDING a partner who is nurturing and loving is a FORMIDABLE task, but somehow we FIND the right person.

We FORGIVE ourselves, our partners, and our children, for making FOOLISH mistakes. We teach FAIRNESS, as well as the responsibility of FENDING for oneself.

We sometimes FALL SHORT of our expectations, and also accept their FLAWS.

We have great hopes for the FUTURE lives of our children, and FORGIVE them, for our love for them is FOOLPROOF. Our FEELINGS about our children are FOREVERMORE.

Breathe in FONDNESS. . . . Breathe out FULFILLMENT. . . .

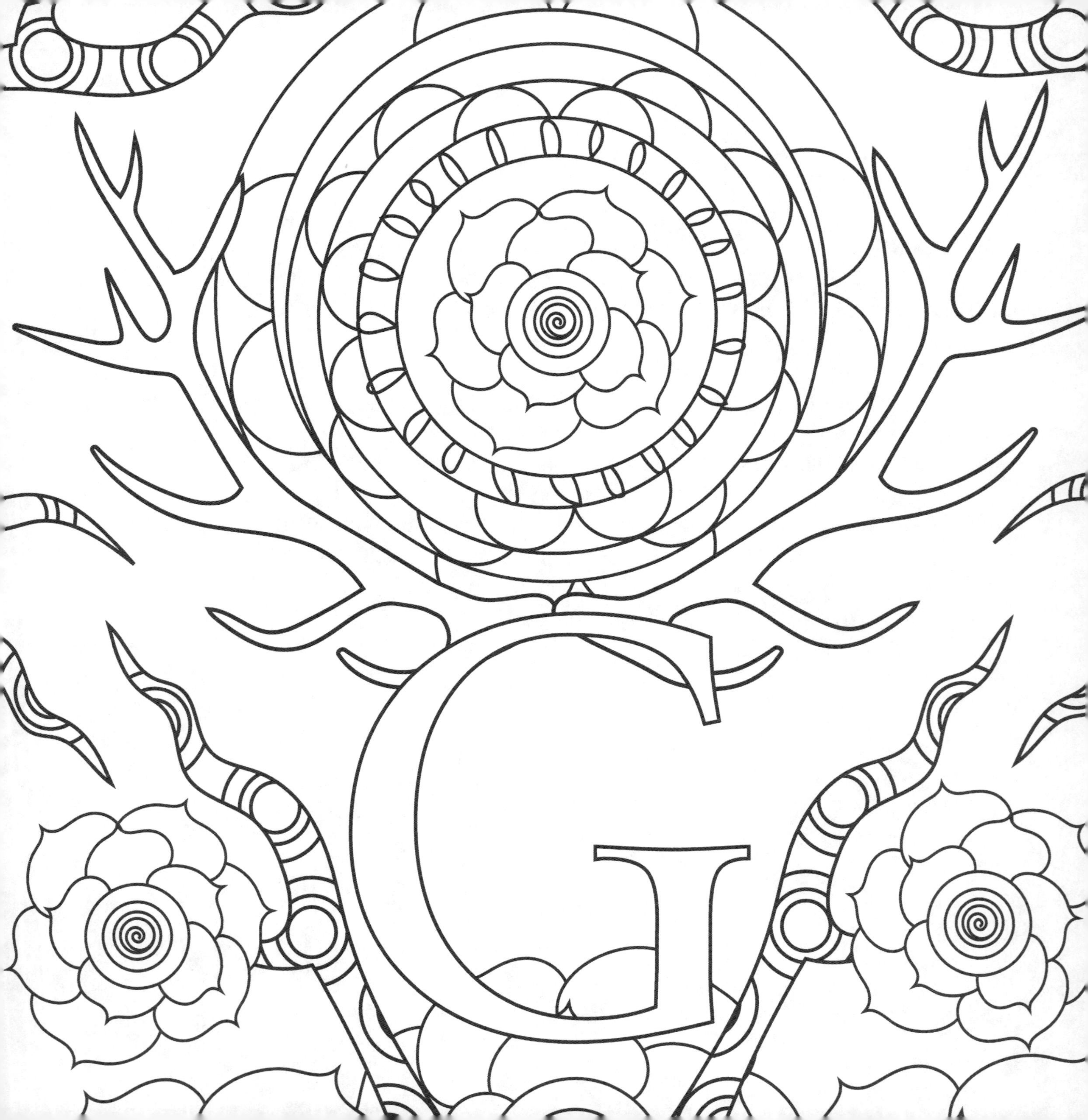
G

G is for GIFT. . . .

Having children is a GIFT from GOD. We GIVE ourselves GREATLY to insure they GROW up to become happy and responsible GOOD people. We think our children are GORGEOUS, and they are, to us.

No matter what GENDER they choose, we support and give them GUIDANCE.

We hope to give them GRACE when dealing with life. Mothers are GODDESSES! We nurture and care for our children's GROWTH. We GOVERN them and GUIDE them through their lives.

GRAPPLING for the right way to teach them about life, we GATHER as much information as we can to GUIDE them.

We GAIN so much from the Motherhood experience, and GENERATE love and wisdom to our children's lives.

We GIVE of ourselves unselfishly and GAIN so much in the process. We are GRACE under pressure, and take nothing for GRANTED. We GO forth in GOODNESS, and are GENEROUS with our time and attention.

Breathe in GRATEFULNESS. . . . Breathe out GOODNESS. . . .

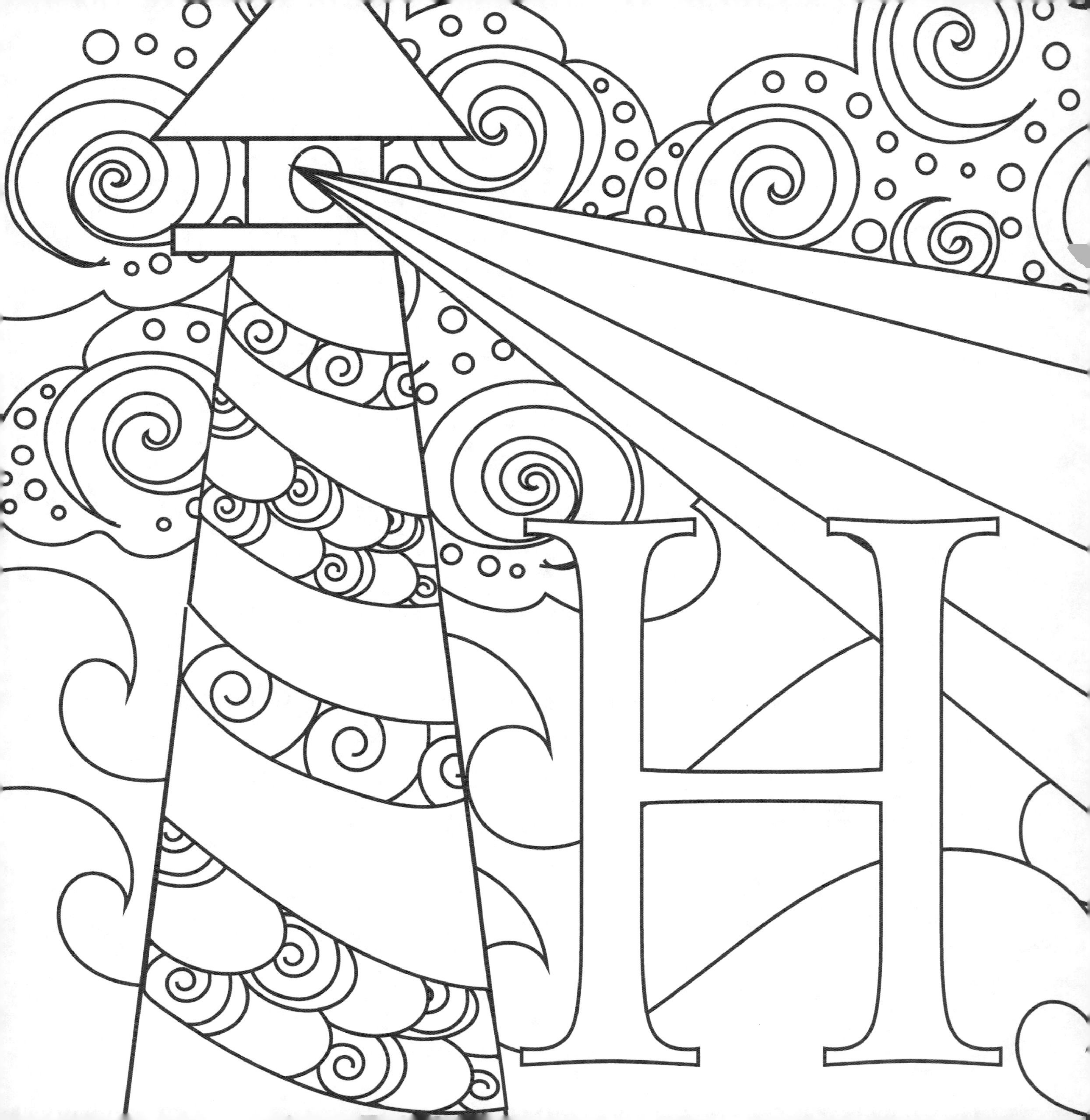
H

H is for HAPPINESS. . . .

The HOURS we share with our children HELP us learn about ourselves. We HONOR their presence in our lives and HOPE to enlighten them.

We HOLD our principles HIGHLY, and try to instill good HABITS that will serve them throughout their lives.

When bad things HAPPEN, we HEAL them with our love and understanding.
Their HEALTH, both physical and mental, is our HEARTFELT priority.

We HUMBLY accept the responsibility of parenting, and we hope to be their HEROES. Our HOMES are their comfort zone.

Breathe in HEALING. . . . Breathe out HOPEFULNESS. . . .

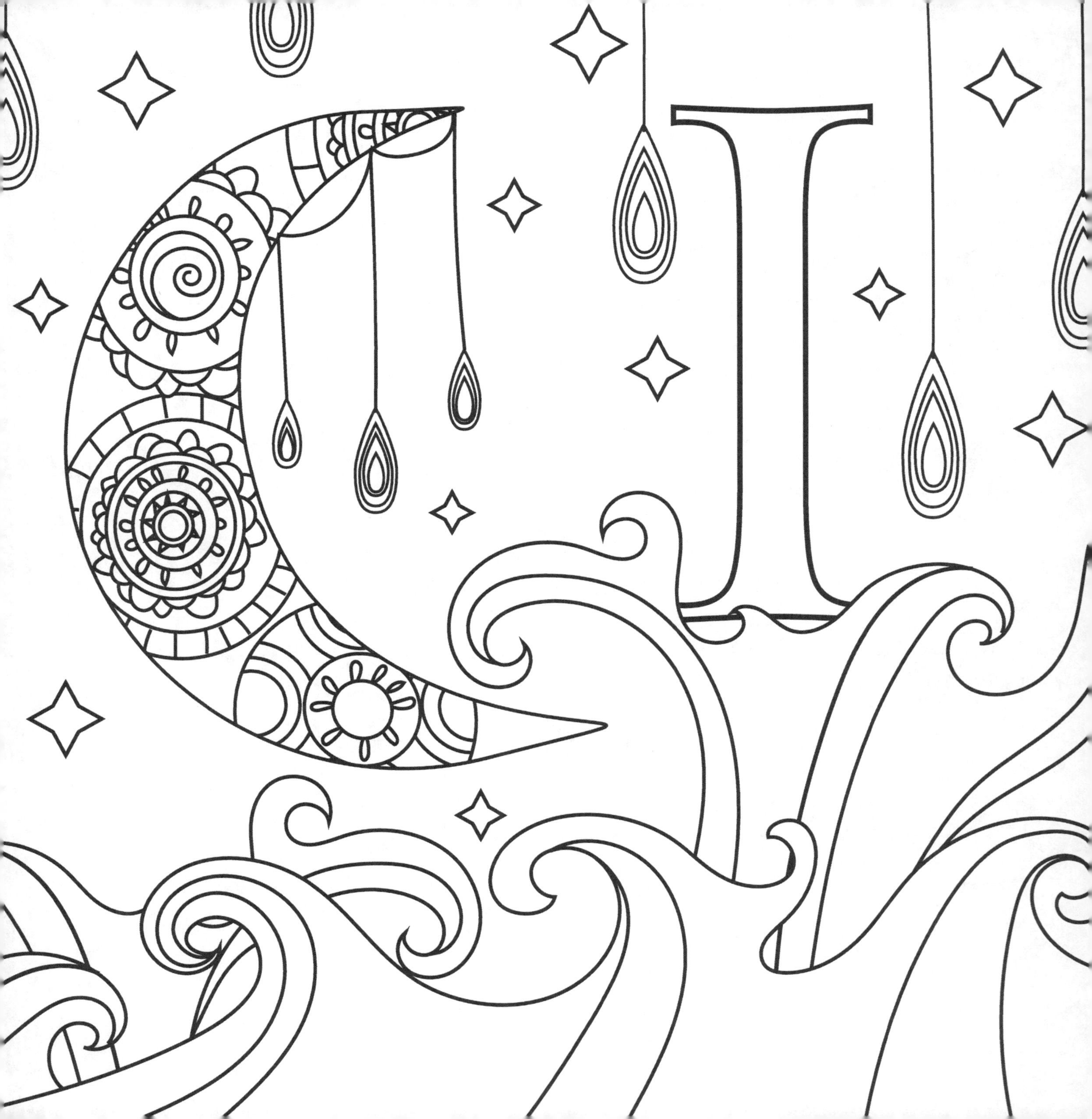

I is for INVINCIBLE. . . .

We want to raise INDEPENDENT children, and strive to teach them to be INTOLERENT of INJUSTICES of any kind.

"IGNORE INAPPROPRIATE behavior" is one of the many lessons I've tried to INSTILL in their lives.

We nurture their INDOMITABLE spirit, and hope that they become IMPERVIOUS and IMMUNE to the negative things that might stand in their path of INNER growth.

We will always try to INFLUENCE them to make INFORMED but INDEPENDENT opinions, and hope that their IMAGINATIONS have no limit to what they can achieve.

We want them to lead INTERESTING lives, and to INCLUDE a spiritual outlook that comforts and INSPIRES them .

Breathe in IMMUNITY. . . . Breathe out IGNORANCE of any kind. . . .

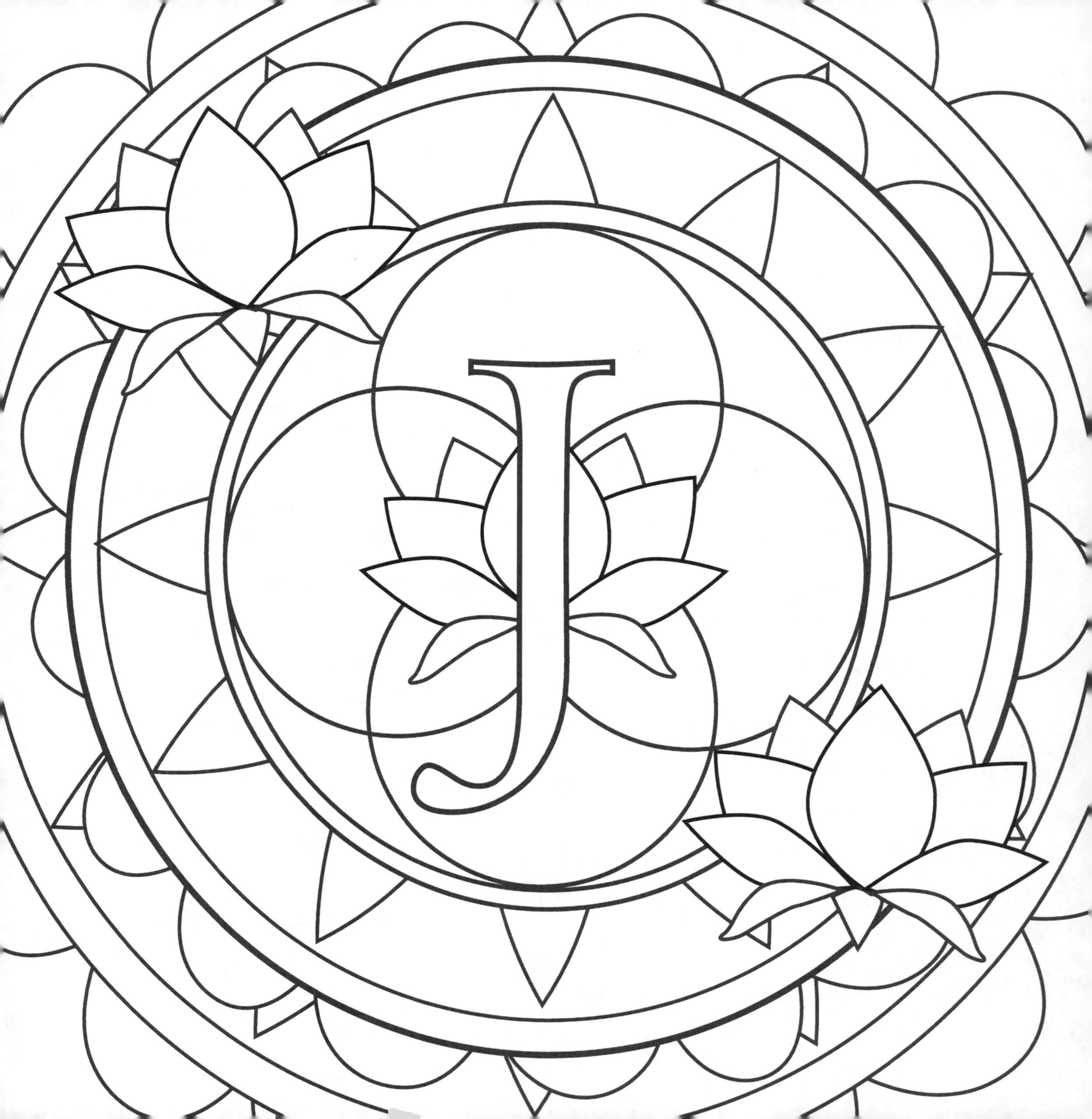
J

J is for JOY. . . .

Motherhood is the most important JOURNEY we take throughout our lives. It is filled with JOYOUS moments as well as JEOPARDIES.

We will try to instill a JOIE DE VIVRE in their spirits, and comfort them when JEALOUSIES arise and JAR their sense of self.

We will enjoy JUBILANT celebrations of their excellence, and sometimes experience JOLTS when life throws its curveballs.

We will try not to be too JUDGEMENTAL, and will be JUDICIOUS in teaching them right actions.

Motherhood is a JUGGLING act. There will be many JUNCTURES where we will teach them wisdom.

Breathe in a sense of JUSTICE. . . . Breathe out JOYFULNESS. . . .

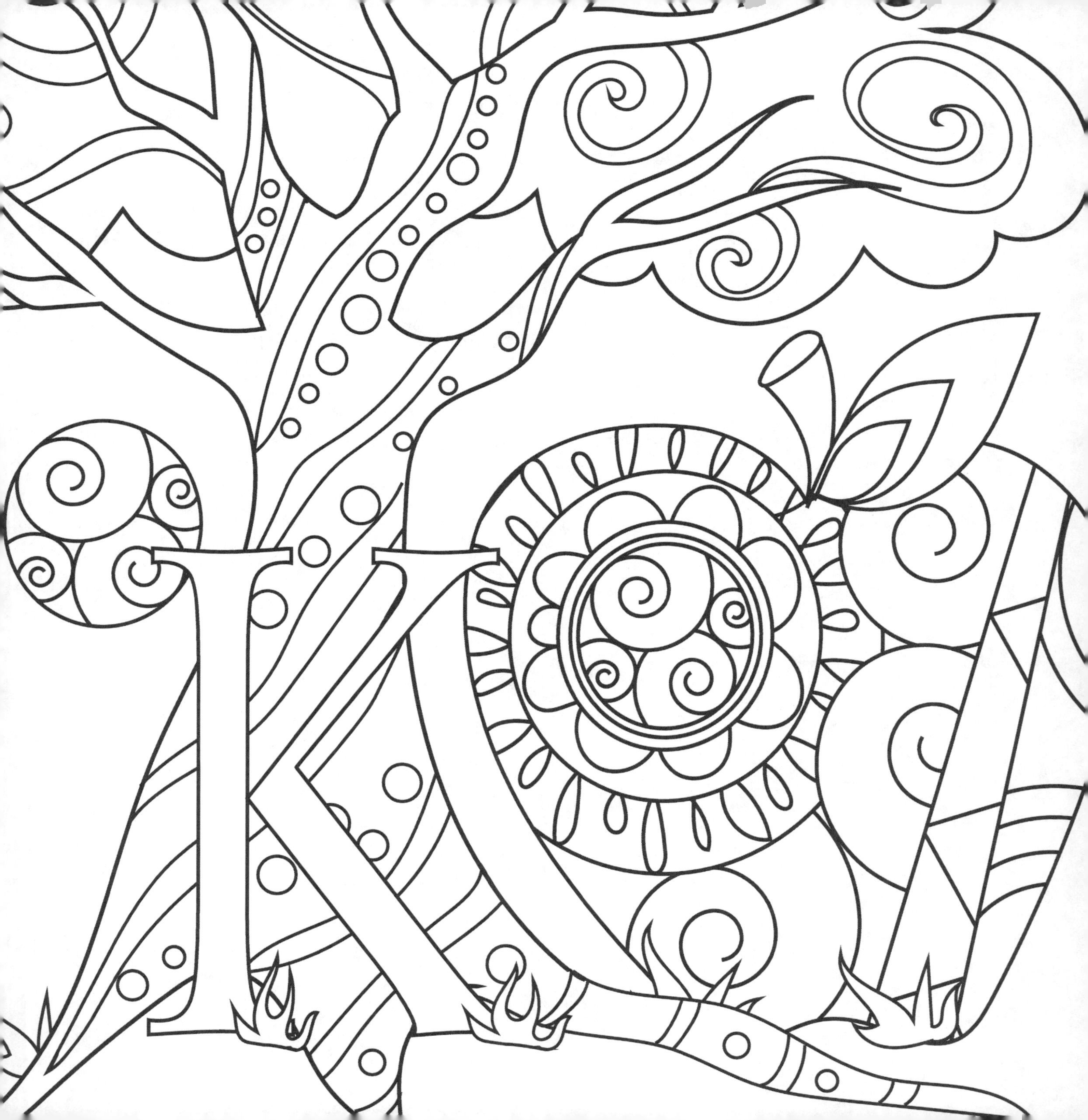
K

K is for KUDOS. . . .

Congratulations on your decision to be a KIND and caring Mother. To KNOWINGLY take on the responsibilities of Motherhood, is a tribute to you.

Yes, Motherhood is full of hard KNOCKS, when you realize you can only direct your children's life, and not the outcome.

A good Mother will instill the lessons of good KARMA, and teach your children to realize that their actions mean something.

A good Mother will be introducing her children to many new interests throughout their developing years, from seeing KANGAROOS at the zoo, to waiting for them during their KARATE lessons.

You hope that they will make a KINGDOM of good friends.

Breathe in KINDNESS. . . . Breathe out KISSES!

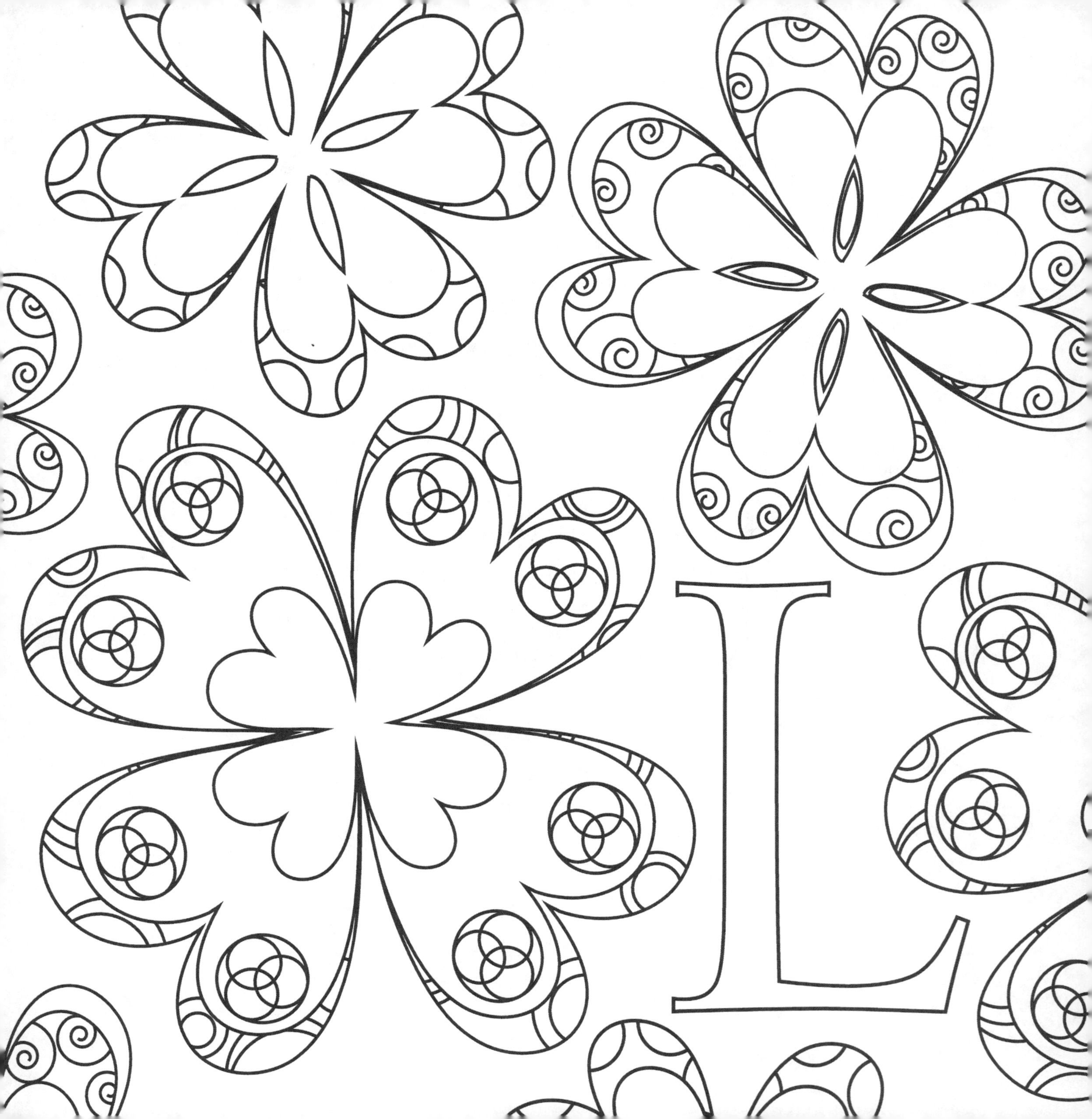
L

L is for LIFE....

As Mothers, we will always be connected to giving our children their LIVES. We start caring for them before they are born by LEARNING to take care of our bodies while they are starting to grow and thrive.

LABOR is not easy, but worth the pain to see our infants LEAVE to inhabit life for themselves. When they are LITTLE, they need us to sustain and nurture themselves.

We LISTEN to their needs, as they grow and become independent people. Part of parenting is learning to LET go, and help them separate from us.

We LEAD them to become the best people they can, and give them unconditional LOVE.

Breathe in LONGING. . . . Breathe out LIBERATION. . . .

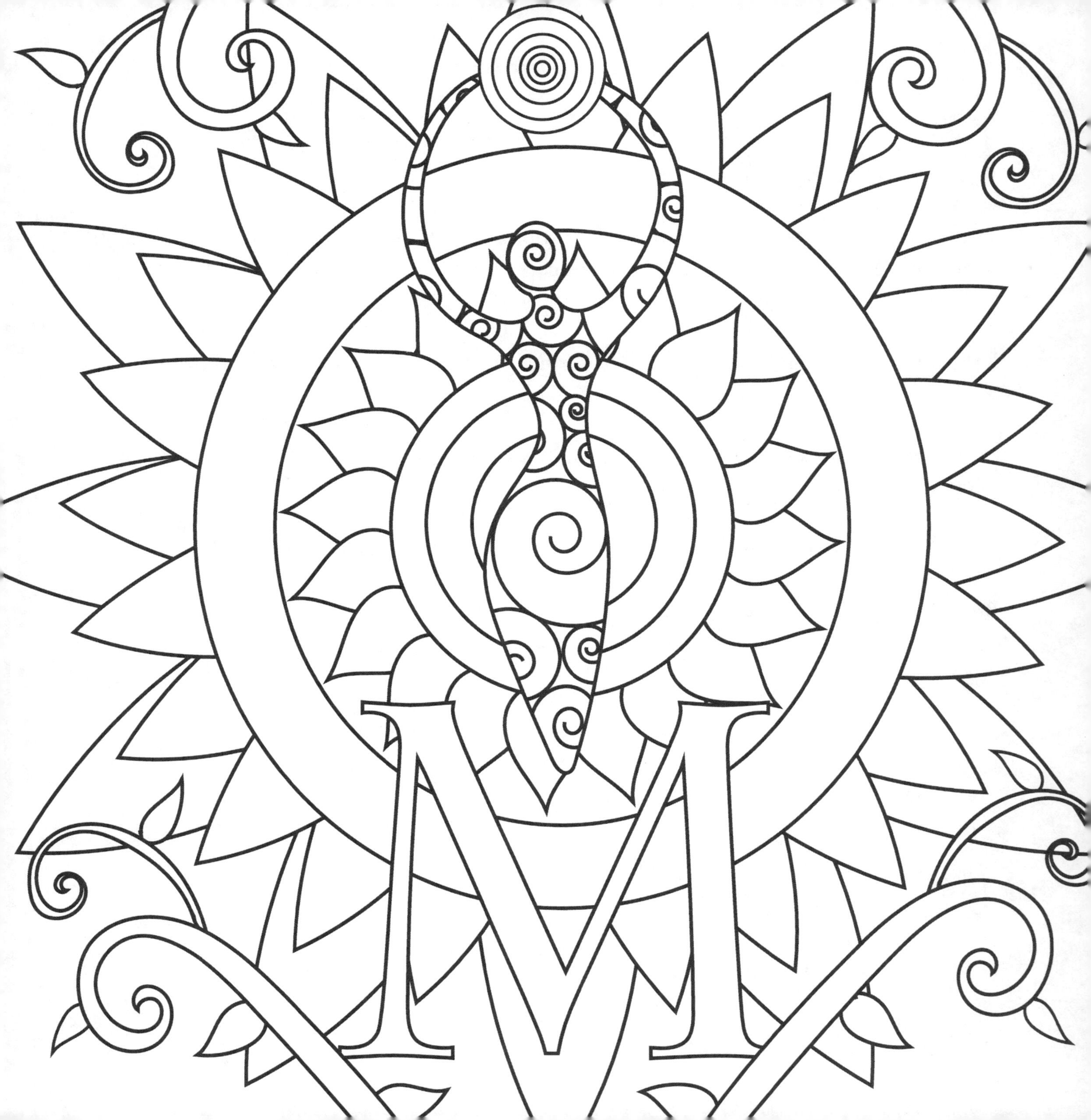
M

M is for MOTHER. . . .

What is the definition of that word? To care for, bring up, love, and nurture—that is the MEANING of MOTHERHOOD.

We try to MAKE our children's lives MAGNIFICENT. We MENTOR them and try to make life MEANINGFUL.

MEMORIES of our Mothers stay with us forever. We want them to enjoy life, and at the same time, teach them MODERATION in all things.

Our children often make our hearts MELT, by their unique expressions and actions.
We hope that they are MENSCHES.

Breathe in MIRACLES. . . . Breathe out MEDITATIONS. . . .

N

N is for NURTURE. . . .

NNURTURING is our role as Mothers—it comes easily, as we NESTLE with our infants in the first few months of life. They NEED us to care for them, and it's a NOBLE yet sometimes demanding task.

We teach them to be NICE, NEVER to lie, and to be kind to one's NEIGHBORS. Mothers are NECESSARY to comfort them in the NIGHT when they hear unfamiliar NOISES.

We give them limits, and have to say NO once in a while. We laugh with them at NONSENSE, and NOURISH them with good NUTRITION.

We hope to instill in them the power of NOW, to be in the moment and enjoy every minute of life.

Breathe in NATURE. . . . Breathe out NECESSITY. . . .

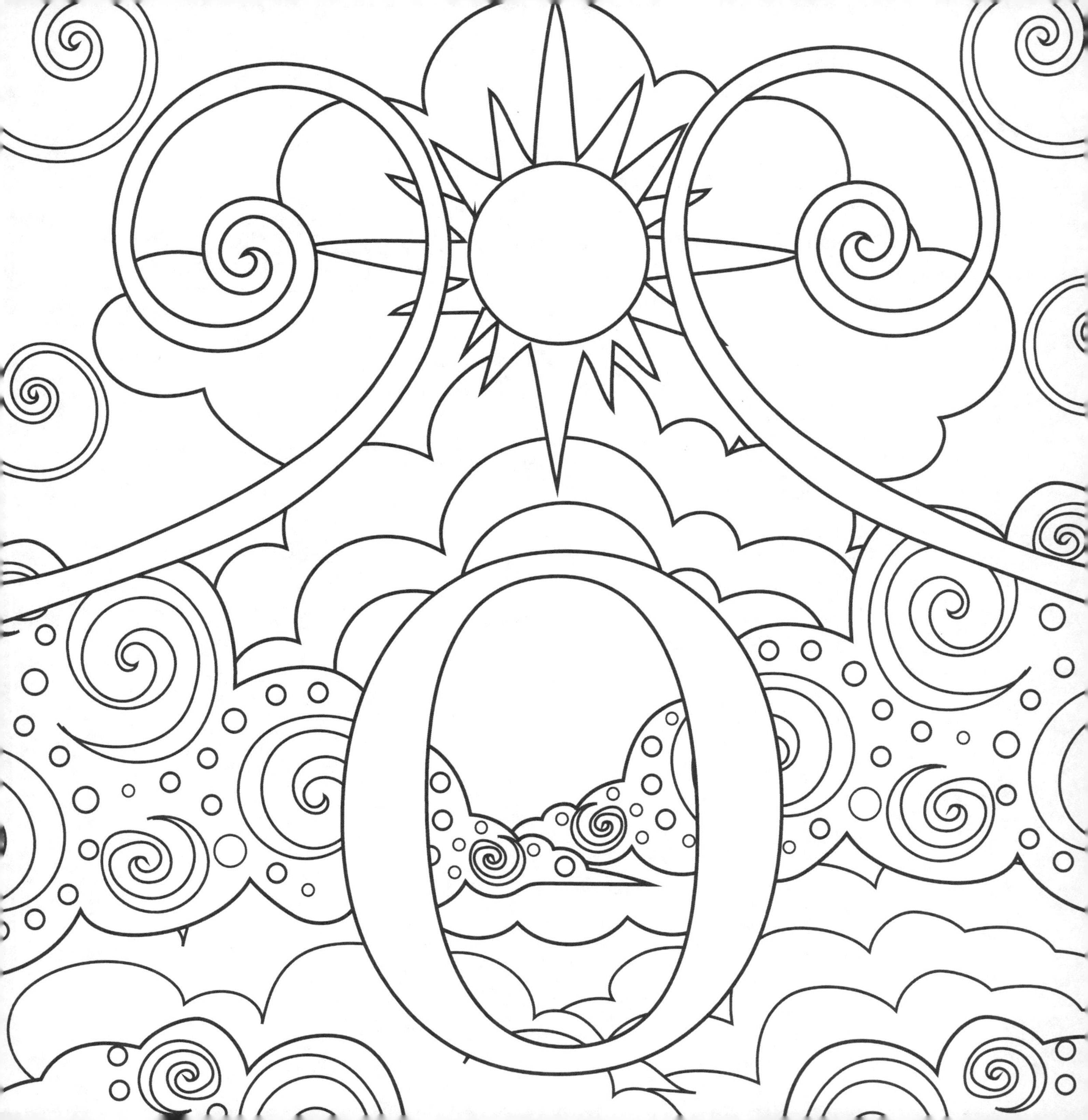
O

O is for OWNERSHIP. . . .

We do not OWN our children. . . . we just borrow them for a time until they can live independently from us.

We are Mothers for ONLY a short time—childhood goes by so fast. We are OBLIVIOUS to the fact that at some point, they will grow away from us, which is the natural ORDER of things.

We OBJECT to inappropriate behavior, and they must OBEY certain limits that we place to keep them happy and safe, to give them OPTIMUM pleasure in life.

We try not to OFFEND their sense of independence, yet at the same time must OFFER our wise counsel.

We let them know they are OKAY, with the choices that come naturally to them, hoping that they will help us when we become OLD.

Breathe in OPENESS. . . . Breathe out OM. . . .

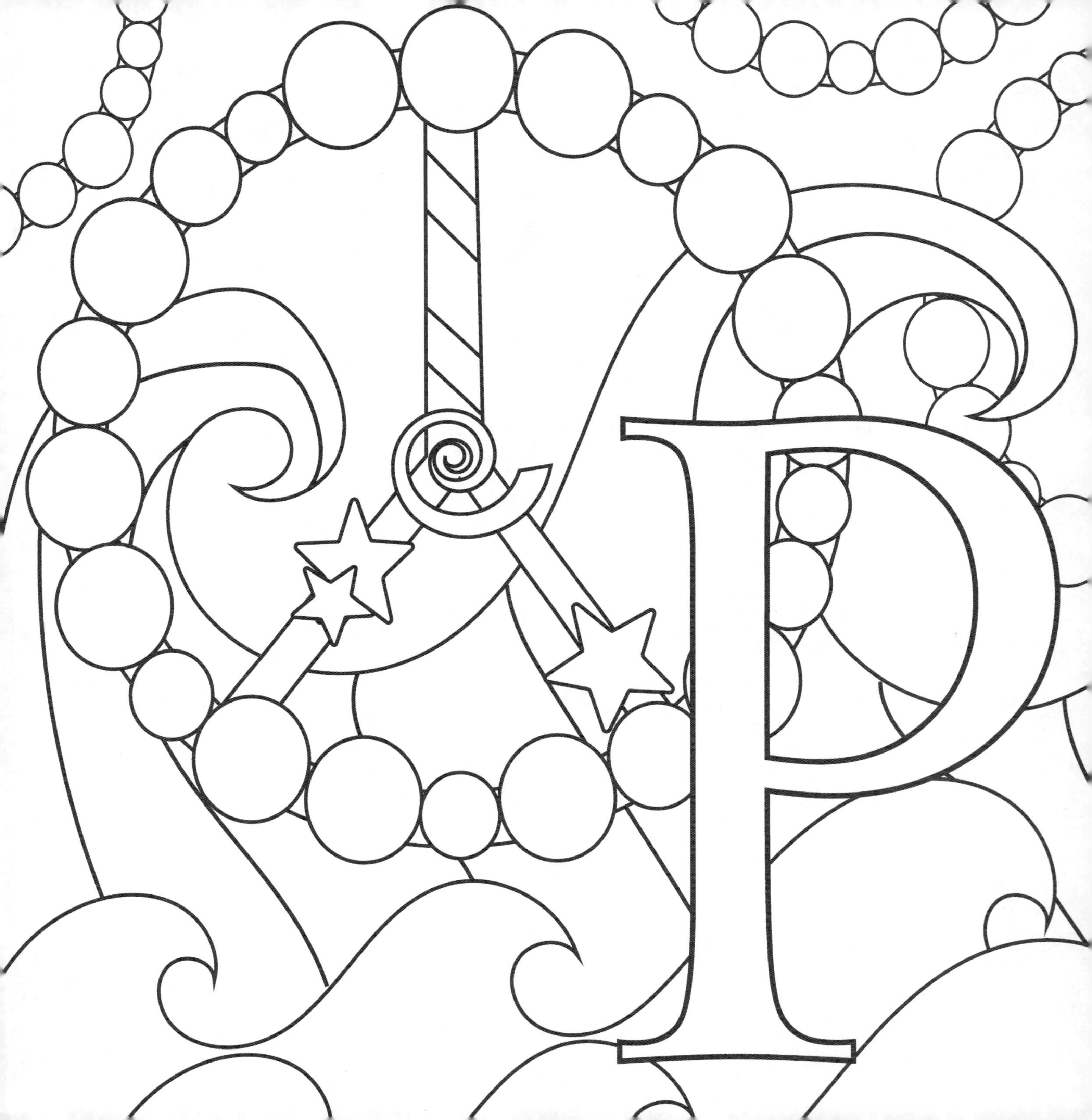
P

P is for PLEASING. . . .

Mother's spend much of their lives trying to PLEASE their children and make their lives wonderful. We are PARTNERS in life and share its ups and downs. We POUR our efforts into making life wonderful for them.

We PROTECT them at all costs, and PRIOITIZE our lives with their needs. We reason with them and try to share our POINTS of view. We PLAY with them and understand their PAIN.

We PRAISE them when they deserve it, and teach them POISE and grace. We PUT things in PERSPECTIVE, and help them POLISH their social skills

When our children are upset, we PACIFY them and comfort their PAIN. We become their PILLARS of strength.

Breathe in PURPOSE. . . . Breathe out PEACE. . . .

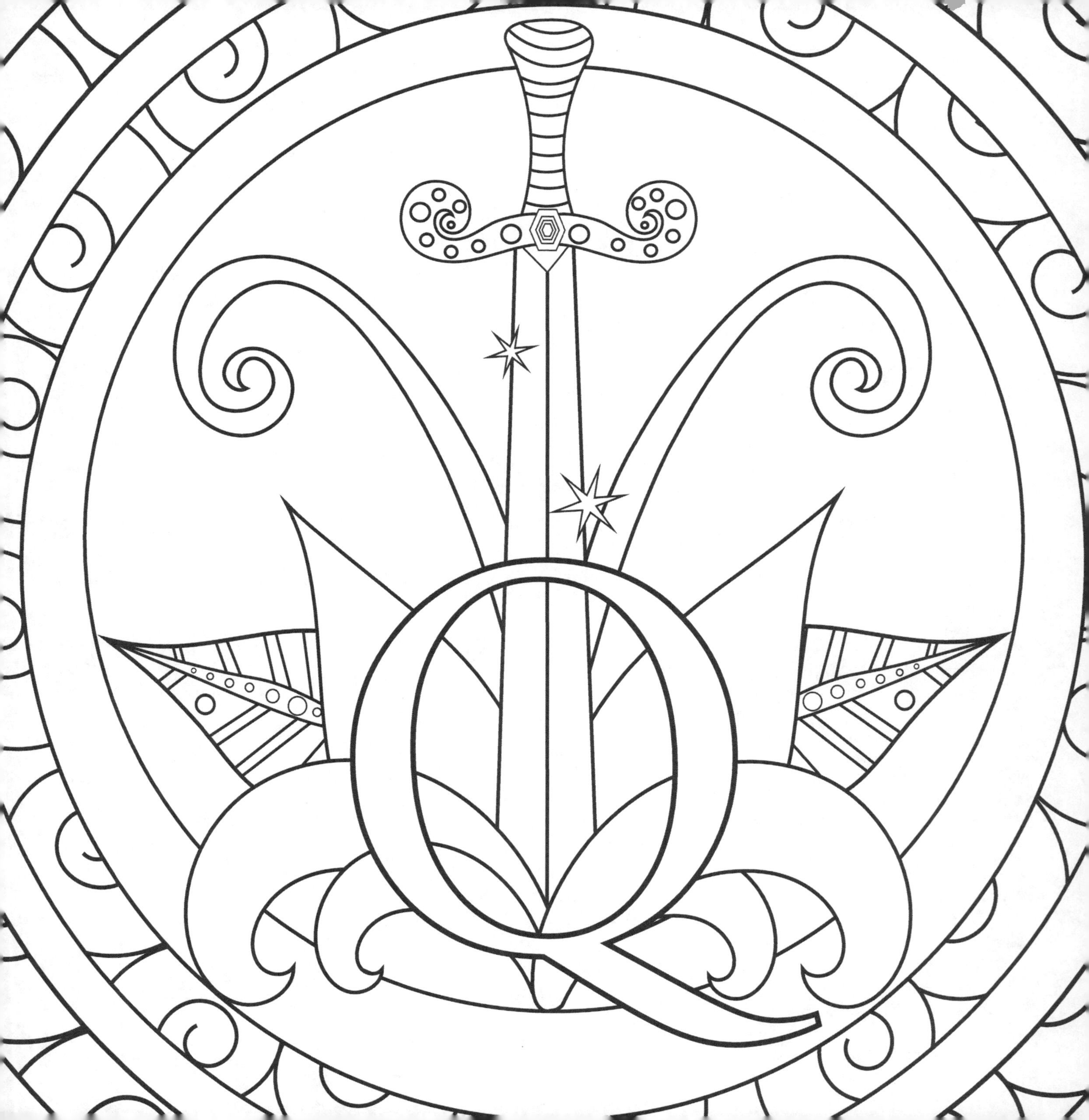

Q is for Quest. . . .

Motherhood is a quest, a search for meaning in our lives. We QUESTION our decisions, actions, and QUALITIES, to make sure we are raising healthy and happy children.

Our QUOTAS are how many days our children are content. We continually ask ourselves if we are QUALIFIED to raise our children well.

We hope to be the QUEEN in their lives, until a partner replaces us, as it should be.

We try to not judge our children too QUICKLY, and put much thought into how to nurture their growth.

Our children are our QUINTESSENTIAL joy.

Breathe in QUALITY. . . . Breathe out QUIETNESS. . . .

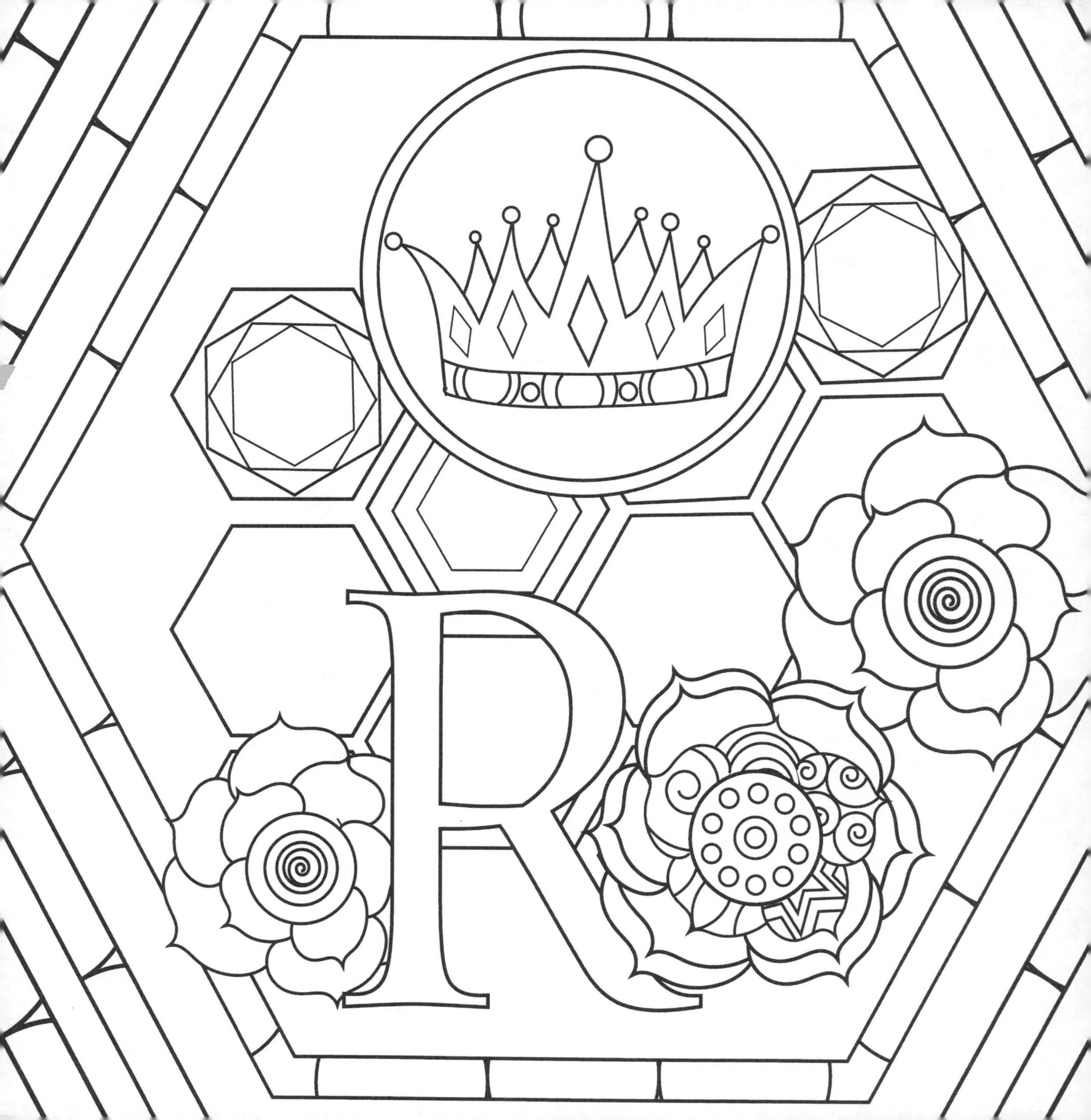

R is for RESOURCEFUL. . . .

As Mothers, we use our RESOURCES to keep our children happy and thriving. We must be RESILIENT and RECTIFY any dangerous situations. We REMAIN Mothers until our deaths, and never RESIST the challenge of being a good parent.

Our children give us a REASON for living, and we RESOLVE to be the best parent we can be. We are RESPONSIBLE for them always, and we RELY on our instincts to protect and nurture them.

We teach them never to be RUDE, and give them RULES to live by. We teach them to be RIGHTEOUS, and to never RUN away from their RESPONSIBILITIES.

We steer them away from RISKY behavior, and ask them to RISE above bad behavior. We are their ROCKS throughout their lives.

Breathe in REASSURANCE. . . . Breathe out REFINEMENT and REFLECTION. . . .

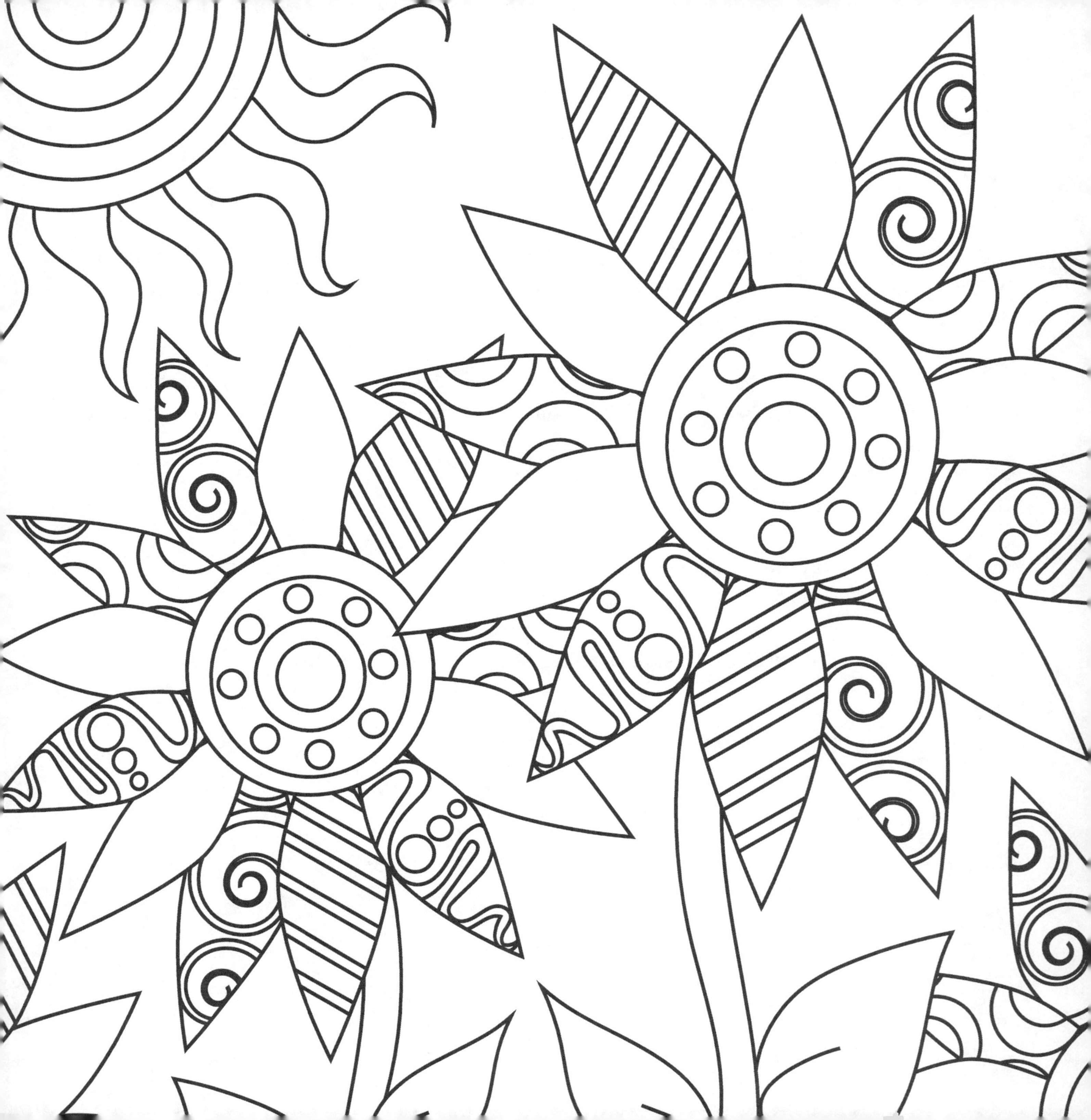

S is for SMILES. . . .

Our children give us SO much joy. They SURPRISE us all the time and SATIATE us with their love. We teach them not to be SELFISH, and try to STIMULATE their interests in the world around them.

We love the SCENTS of babies—they SATISFY us when they are happy. Our needs are SECOND to theirs and we strive to make them feel SECURE. They SEDUCE us with their laughter and we SEIZE all the joy we can from them.

We teach them SELF-RESPECT and hope that they grow in a SELFLESS manner. Although we must SEPARATE from them as they grow, we hope, as we become SENIORS, they will cherish us.

We SPEND time with them, and teach them SILLY words and phrases.

Breathe in SACRIFICE. . . . Breathe out SUPPORTIVE. . . .

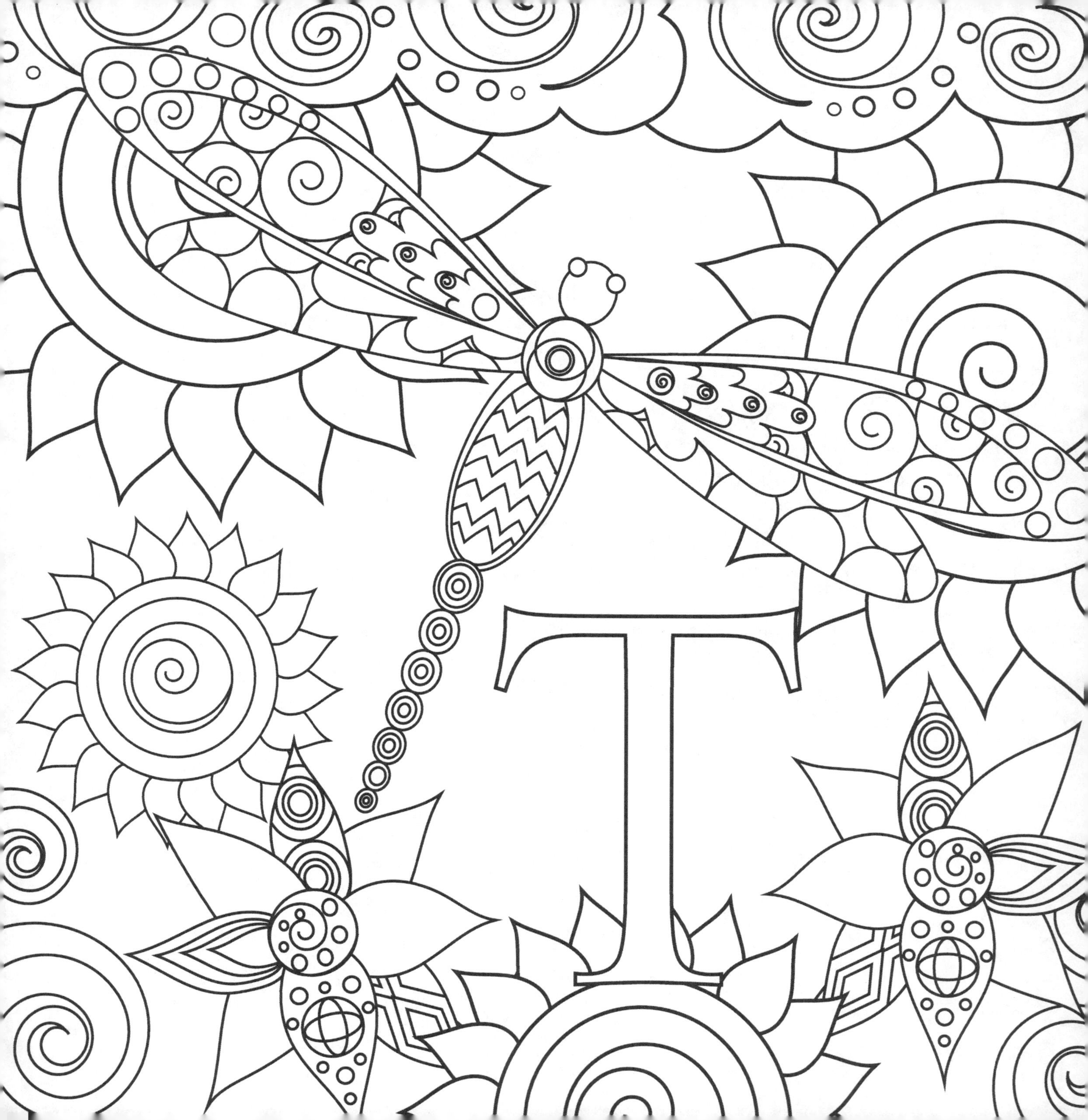
T

T is for TRIUMPHANT. . . .

Being a Mother is our greatest TRIUMPH—we TEACH our children everything we can to make THEM flourish. There will be TEARS of sorrow, and of joy, as we raise them with our love.

We TELL them again and again, how to navigate the TRENCHES that life offers.

We TUCK them in every night, and TICKLE them to hear their laughter. We watch them grow as TODDLERS, and hug them TIGHTLY.

Our greatest gift is TIME. We dry their TEARS with TISSUES, and tell them to believe in the TOOTH Fairy. We give them the life TOOLS they need, and even when they are TIMID, we encourage them to deal with TURMOIL.

Even though sometimes we are TIRED, we TUNE out our needs and take care of them.

Breathe in THANKFULNESS. . . . Breathe out TOLERANCE. . . .

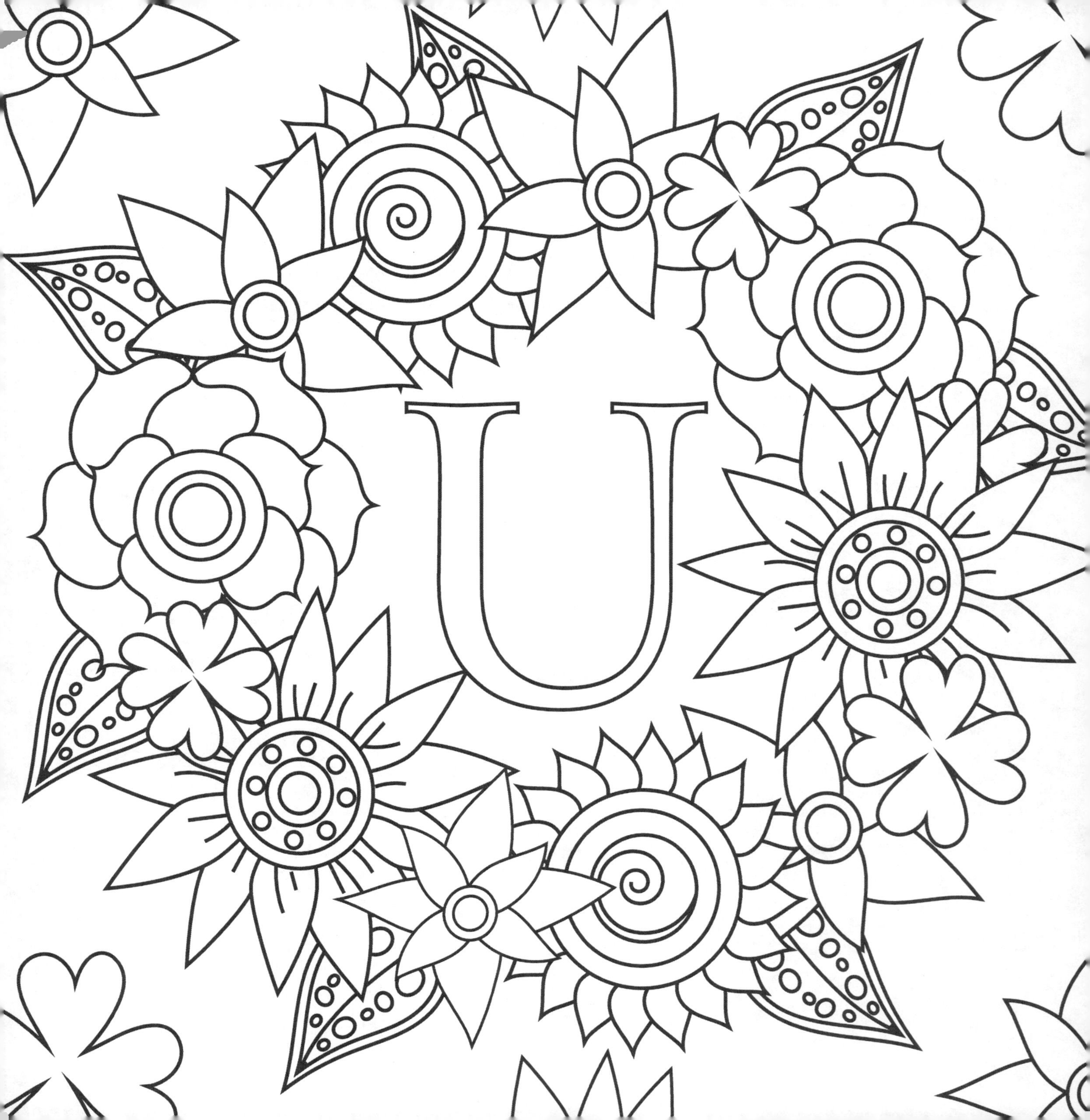
U

U is for UNDERSTANDING. . . .

We sometimes UNDERESTIMATE our children. We are UNITED, in wanting what is best for them, but at the same time struggle to UNDERSTAND their needs.

Each and every child is UNIQUE, and we are their UMBRELLAS, as we shelter them.

They are our UNCHARTED territory, and we love them UNABATEDLY and know that our love for them is ULTIMATE.

We do not stand for UNJUSTNESS in their lives, and we are UNAMUSED when someone bullies them—it is simply UNACCEPTABLE.

We are their UMPIRES in the game of life. At times, we are unappreciated, but our love stays UNBOUNDED.

Breathe in UNCERTAINTY. . . . Breathe out USEFULNESS. . . .

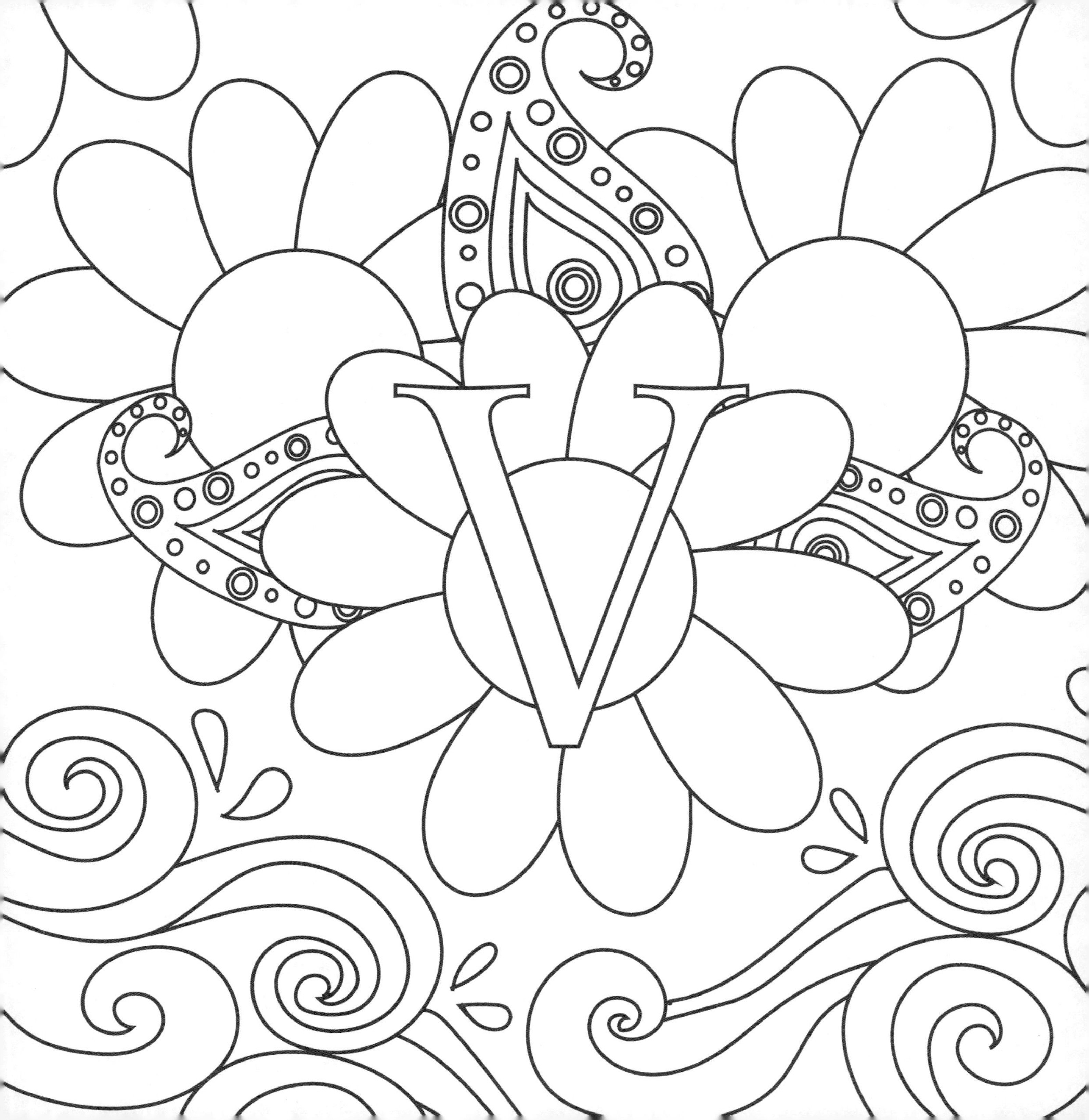
V

V is for VICTORIOUS. . . .

We score a VICTORY when our children are happy. We teach them the power of VIRTUE, as well as VIVACIOUSNESS.

Our children are VIBRANT, and move at VELOCITIES that astound us. We sometimes have to VIE for their attention, and always treasure their VALUE in our lives.

Our emotions sometimes VACILLATE, as we observe their VULNERABILITES.

We take them on VACATIONS to show them the world. It can feel like a VORTEX when we are in the room with their high energies.

We hope to teach them not to be VAIN, and to keep a check on their VANITY.

Breathe in VALUABLE. . . . Breathe out VIGILANCE. . . .

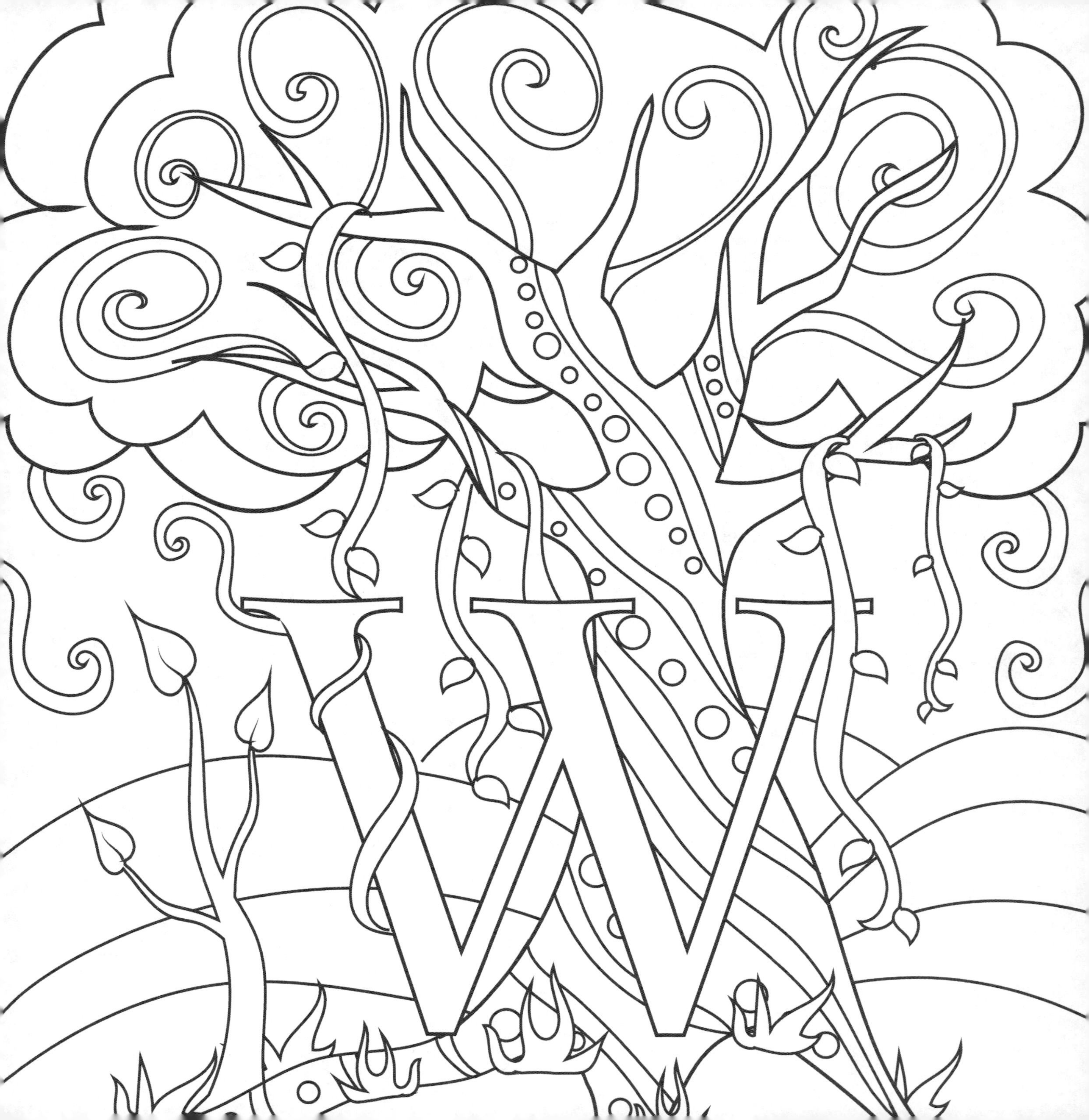
W

W is for WONDERMENT . . . .

WOMEN are nurturers by nature. WE WANT the best for our children, and WORRY about them throughout our lives.

We pave the WAY for them to mature and lead WONDERFUL lives. We WAIT for them to comprehend the meaning of their lives, as we teach them to WIN when they can, but not to WALLOW in their failures.

We teach them to WALK on WOBBLY legs, and WHISPER gentle encouragements, as they become WHO they were meant to be. We try to instill a sense of WONDER about life and the universe.

We teach them the meaning of WHY?

Breathe in WORTHY. . . . Breathe out WELLNESS. . . .

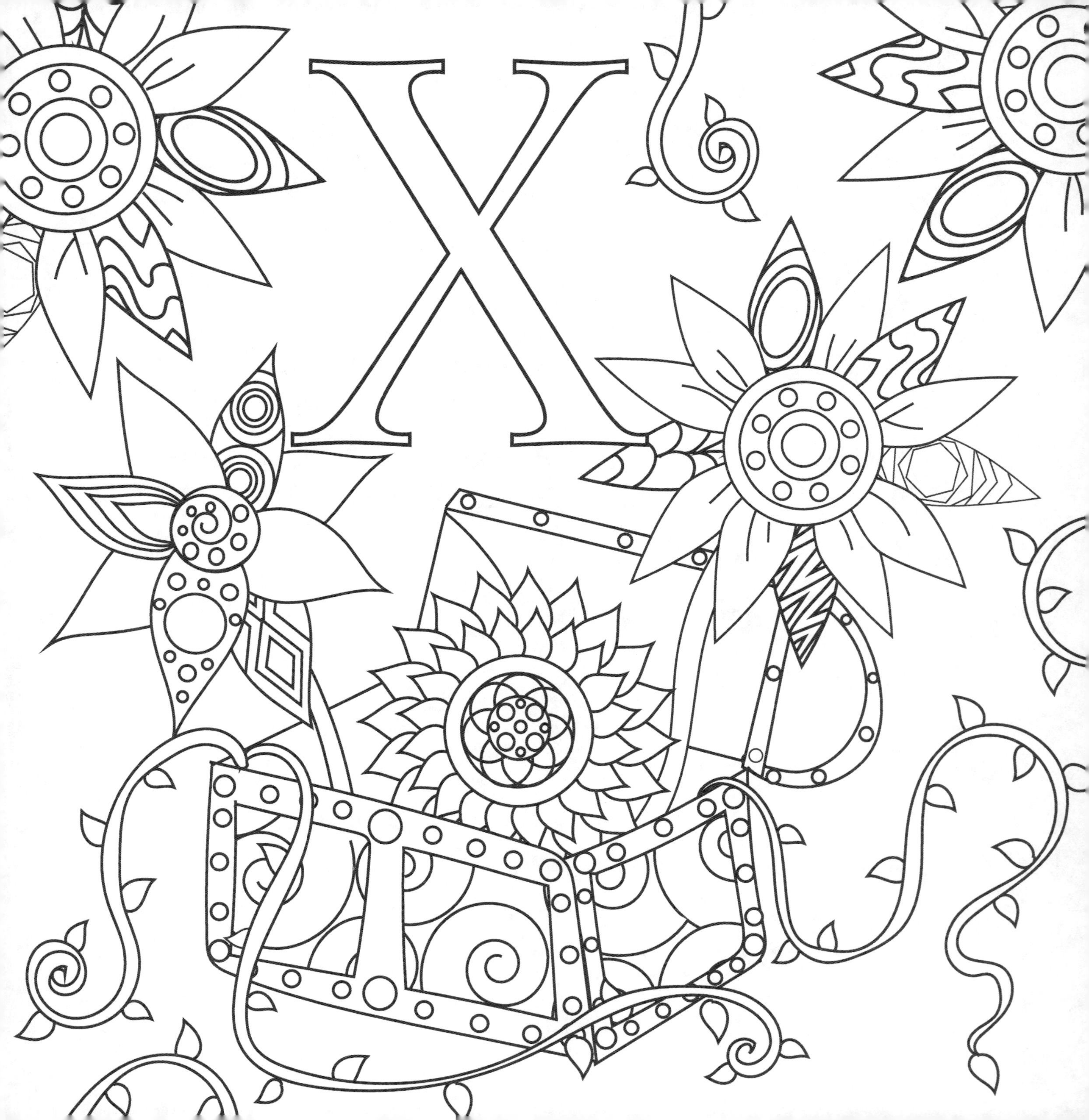
X

X is for you to create your hopes and dreams on this page for your children!.

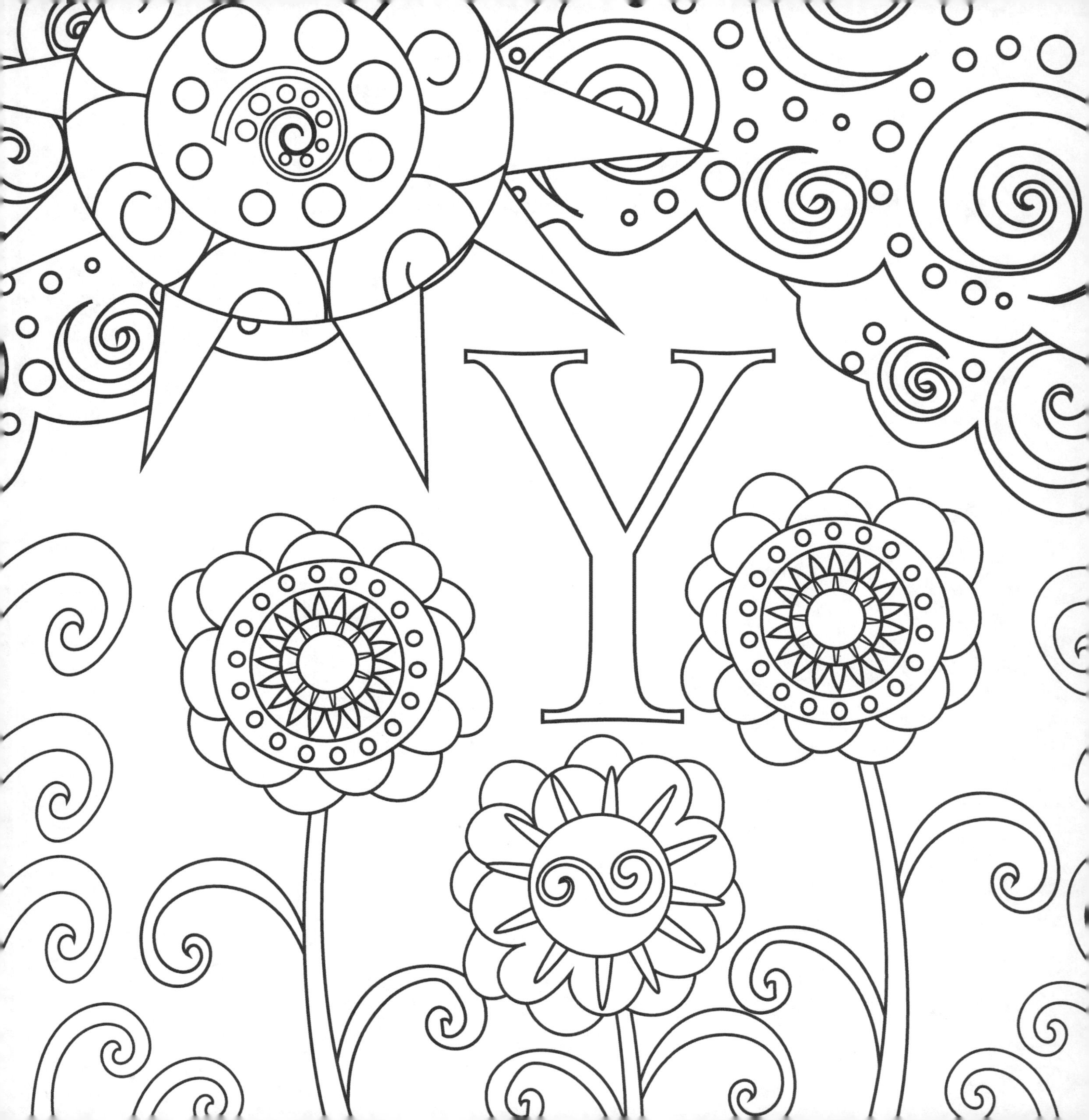
Y

Y is for YOU!

YOU have decided on being a Mother for all the YEARS of YOUR life. When our children are YOUNG, we YEARN to nurture and protect them.

We sometimes YIELD to their whims to keep them happy. We teach them fun words like YAHOO and YIPPEE!

We might introduce them to YOGA. We must keep in mind that YOUTH flies by, and all our moments will someday be YESTERDAY.

In bringing up your children, you must learn to also be gentle with YOURSELF. No Mother is perfect, and we sometimes act in YUCKY ways!

Breathe in YEARNING. . . . Breathe out YES!!!!

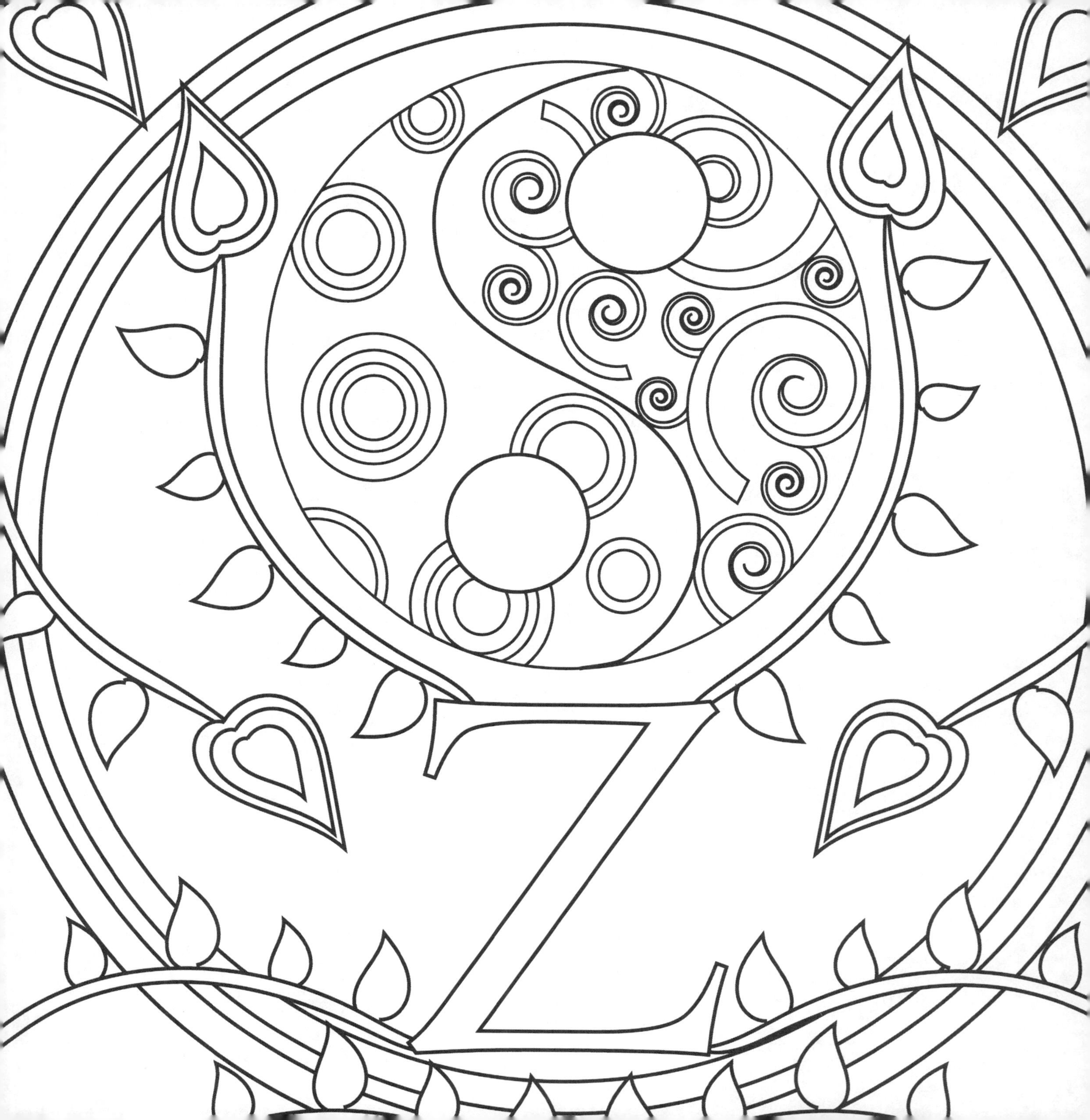
Z

Z is for ZEALOUS. . . .

We ZEALOUSLY raise our children, and hope they have ZERO problems in their life.

When they do encounter life's challenges, we teach them to be ZEN-LIKE, and to ZIG-ZAG around them.

We hope they become ZILLIONAIRES, but teach them humility. We tell them about the ZODIAC, and take them to the ZOO.

We might teach them to dance the ZUMBA, and to enjoy the ZEST for life and ZABAGLIONE!

Breathe in ZANY. . . . Breathe out ZENITH. . . .

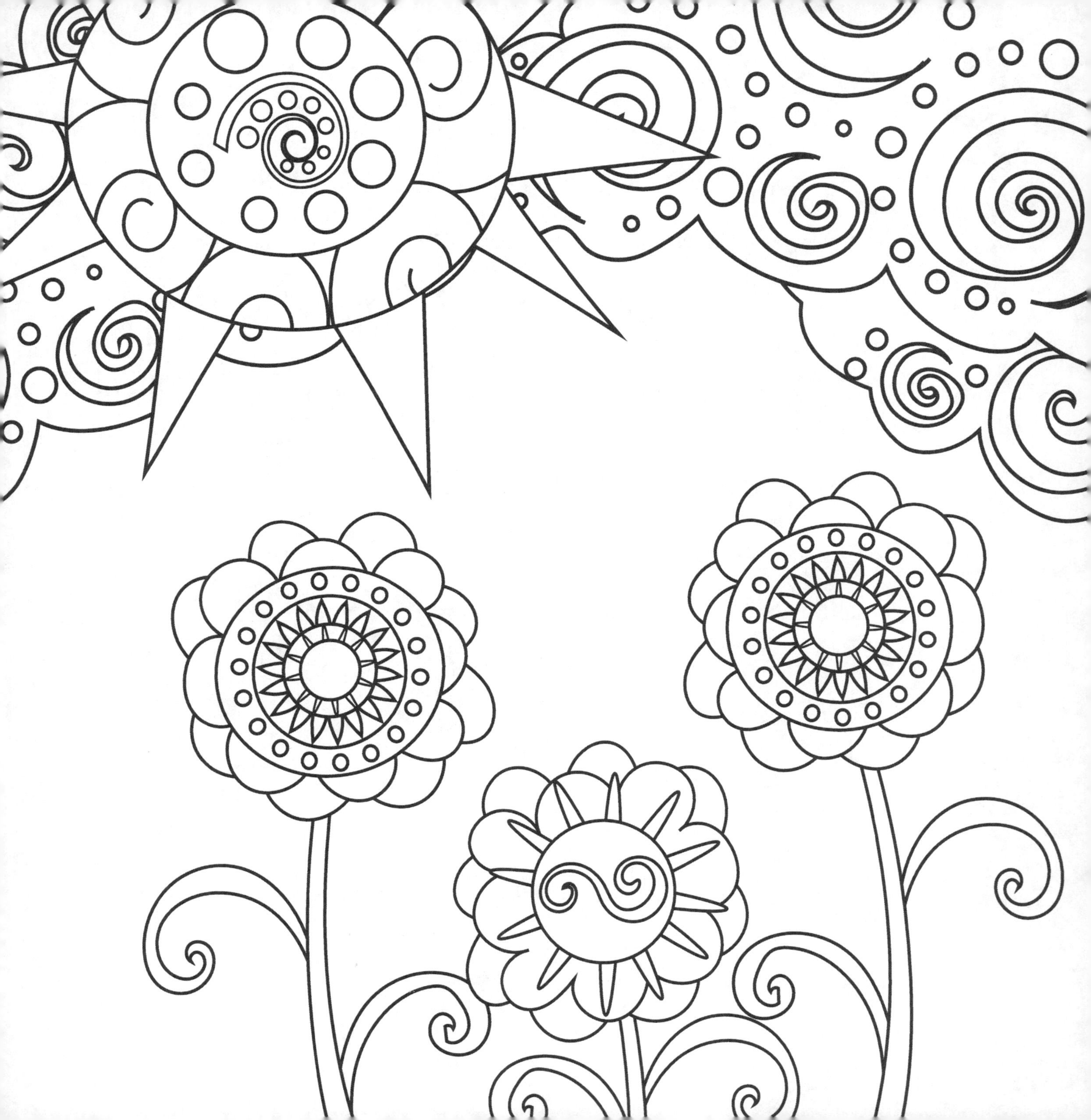

Conclusion

I hope these words have contributed to your joy of experiencing Motherhood. The timing is interesting as I write this conclusion. My own son was married this year and is now expecting a baby boy of his own! Every moment you share is precious, and we continue to enjoy each other's company as we both grow older. I can't wait to watch his own son, my grandchild, grow into the wise and kind person that I know he will raise. Bon chance to all of you in this dance of life! It has been a privilege to share my thoughts on this very special and important relationship.

Namaste,

J. K. Collins

Reputation Books